Sari;
All the best to you
and your family!
With Love,
Pamela

PLANT-BASED DONE RIGHT

HANDBOOK

EAT GRASS, KICK ASS

Pamela Burnham BSN RN

Disclaimer: The information in this book contains the opinions and ideas of its author and is solely intended to provide helpful general information on the subject matter. The subject matter is ever changing the in the world of science and health.
It is not intended to be a substitute for your doctor(s) medical advice. Before you change your diet, whether it be whole food plant-based, vegetarian, vegan, or any other, you should consult with a certified physician and/or other qualified healthcare professional.

This applies to everyone, especially those who have renal or liver disease, are pregnant or may become pregnant, are under the direct care of a physician for any condition, or are on medicine of any kind including and especially insulin, blood thinners, and cardiac medications.

First Edition: May 2021

8 7 6 5 4 3 2

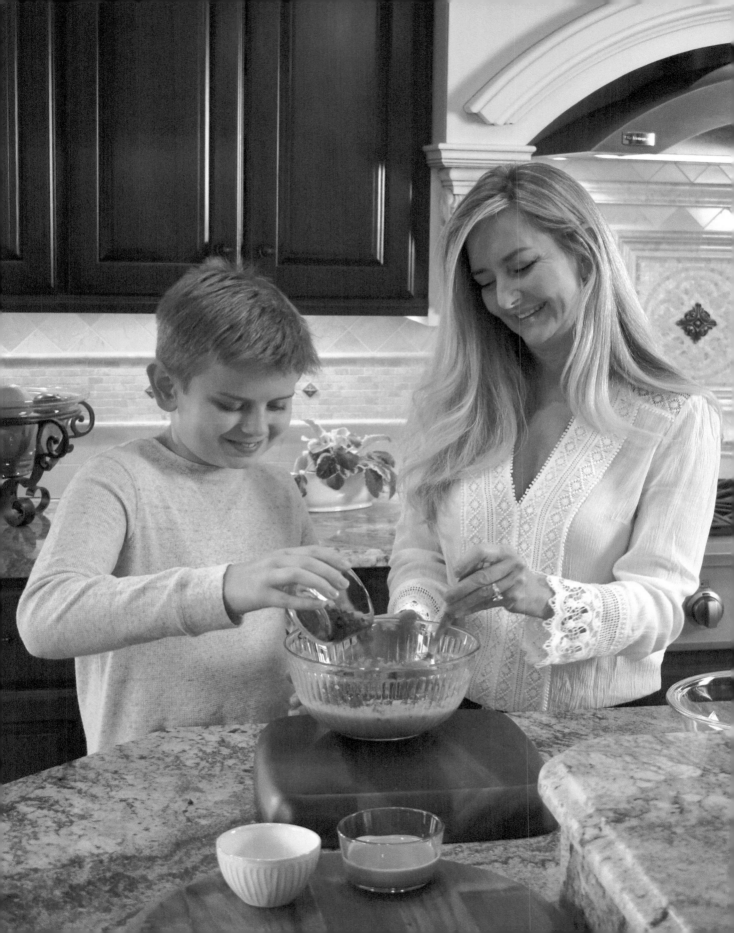

ACKNOWLEDGMENTS

This book is dedicated to many, but especially my husband for his support, encouragement, sacrifice, and hard work that have made it possible for me to write this book; our children Lauren, Heather, and Luke for their continuous desire to learn, their caring and efforts to help others, and for supporting me through this endeavor; my parents for always being there and being supportive in everything I do and providing the best for me and my siblings; my sisters for their support and assistance in editing and being brutally honest when necessary; my military sisters who were a significant influence in many ways and continue to provide healthy and positive support for one another during family separations and difficult times; many friends and patients seeking the truth about health and the nutritional experts and their families who sacrifice so much and spend their lives doing all they can to help others live healthy productive lives.

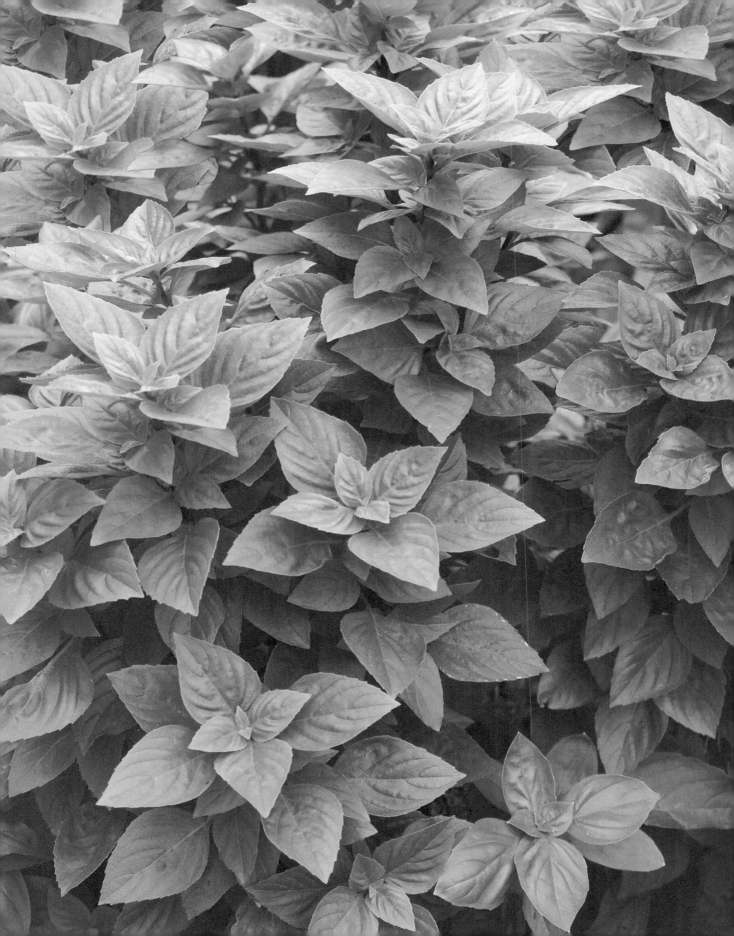

CONTENTS

INTRODUCTION

My Story: Why This Book?

I was born with a heart defect and gastroenteritis so severe that nothing would stay in my stomach. For much of my first year of life, I received my nutrition through IV needles in my ankles. Though I was thin and very active through my growing years, I suffered from irritable bowels, lactose intolerance, various skin allergies, lower back pain, migraine headaches, and crippling hip joint pain. In my teens and into adulthood, I saw that my mom suffered from debilitating health issues too, only hers were worse. She had frequent migraine headaches, severe asthma, arthritic joint pain, Meniere's disease, shingles, severe allergic reactions to nearly every antibiotic and pain medication, gall stones, and spinal cord disk compression. Additionally, my parents ended up on cardiac medications. As my younger sisters grew older, they, too experienced multiple health problems, including thyroid issues, arthritis, and cardiac disease involving silent heart attacks before middle age. I couldn't understand why my family was afflicted with so many disorders, for we have always been a family who loved the land, growing plenty of fruit and vegetables to nourish our bodies. We grew up eating handpicked tomatoes, sweet raspberries, and peas right off the vine. My parents, for whom their garden was a source of pride and joy, tried to set a good example, not only with what they brought to our kitchen table from our garden but also by what they did not bring. My parents were light consumers of beer and wine and smoking was a thing of the past. So why then did we have so many medical problems? Why did I grow up with the stress of worrying that I might one day be as sick or sicker than my parents, living with so many maladies and pain? For years, these questions hounded me. I was determined to do everything I could to outrun a spiraling bullet with my name on it. I was determined to outrun numerous health issues, including high cholesterol, which runs in my family and worsens as we age. I armed myself for my race by eating a mostly vegetarian diet, only occasionally dabbling in fish, chicken, and nonfat dairy products. I avoided fried food and used only extra virgin olive oil, drank a small amount of wine occasionally, rarely ate any dessert, and exercised for nearly an hour every day.

Despite my interventions, as an adult, my total cholesterol levels would surge into the danger zone and doctors recommended I start on cholesterol-lowering medication. The last thing in the world I wanted to do was take medicine for my problems knowing they lead to other disorders as I had seen first hand in my family and as a nurse. Frustrated by my genetics, I continued to fight my battle naturally, hoping to stay out of the pharmacy. One of my many strategies to improve my health included always broiling or baking fish and using only small amounts of virgin olive oil on my food in an attempt to reduce my LDL "bad" cholesterol levels. While this approach certainly raised my HDL "good" cholesterol levels, my total cholesterol levels remained elevated into a risk category that would typically lead to the need to take statins. I preferred to avoid this drug knowing the complications—including the potential for developing diseases such as diabetes, hypothyroidism, or liver problems. Believing the only possible remaining evil remaining in my diet was chocolate, I only allowed myself to eat it once in a while. Though I continued to consume chocolatey food occasionally, I experienced facial redness and hives when I did. Little did I know, however, that my life was about to change and that because of that, those skin problems, cholesterol battles, and other health struggles, including the severe arthritic joint pain, would become history.

My personal evolution, which began in my mid to late forties, was ignited by a new habit incorporated into my morning treadmill routine. Rather than listening to music while exercising, I watched TV and discovered several health-related documentaries with a firm foundational belief in "nutrition as medicine ."

Among my favorites were "Forks over Knives" and "Fat, Sick, and Nearly Dead." Through these documentaries I learned about a new way of eating, an approach referred to as a Whole Food Plant-Based Diet. Initially, I was a huge skeptic about this eating lifestyle, wondering how in the world people were getting enough protein and calcium without consuming any meat or dairy, but the miraculous testimonials and study findings in the documentaries so enthralled me that I couldn't stop thinking or talking about them. I began to seriously wonder if my family's long-running medical mystery could be linked to the fact that, despite all the wonderful fruit and vegetables we had consumed over the years, we had still eaten chicken, fish, egg, and dairy products. We'd always thought this food was healthy, but the documentaries made me question my previously held assumptions. If indeed the key to controlling my impending heart disease and existing problems lay in removing meat, dairy, and eggs from my diet, I was willing to give it a try. But first, I wanted to learn more about the whole food plant-based diet.

I began scooping up every book written by these scientists and doctors who developed the science behind it. I attended every possible conference for which they would be in attendance to hear them speak. This was my new favorite way to earn my continuing education units for maintaining my nursing licensure. As I was learning and trying new food, an extraordinary thing happened when I replaced the dairy products in my chocolate desserts with dairy-free products. My skin problems disappeared. I could eat dairy-free chocolate all day long if I wanted to and "Enjoy Life," one of my first favorite brands of nondairy chocolate chips. Of course, I knew I had to eat a variety of sensible types of food as well. But enjoying pure-cocoa nondairy-milk chocolate-banana shakes without the skin problems thrilled me. Almost instantly, I became a whole food plant-based diet believer though I didn't completely quit eating chicken, fish, eggs, and a few other staples of the Standard American Diet (SAD), mostly because my family still insisted on them. Then I reached a turning point. A surgical procedure forced me to adopt a strict WFPBD for several months, during which time I experienced the positive though drastic changes this way of eating could result in, including dropping weight without effort and recovering quickly from major surgery. I lost nearly twenty pounds, leading me, the mother of three, to a weight I hadn't seen in decades—at five foot two, I was now 112 pounds, and my cholesterol levels had fallen dramatically, settling in at healthy ranges. One of the most amazing things was that I could now eat without restriction, not worry about portion control, and kept the weight off without much effort.

As the life of my body and mind were dramatically changing because of my improved diet, I looked at research studies that definitively showed that many common types of food were negatively affecting my family. This made me particularly concerned for my elementary-age son, who was just getting on the road to better eating habits. The more I learned about the science behind plant-based food and the many ways it improves the body, even when we are in the womb, the more I realized I wanted to immerse not only myself in a whole food plant-based way of life but my family as well. So, after many years of living half in and half out of the WFPBD world, with the exception of the time I was prepping for surgery and in recovery, I began to strictly transition my way of eating and help my family do the same. Initially, it was undoubtedly a challenge. I had to ease my son and my husband, a retired Navy commander who had been as fit as a fiddle in his youth, but had put on nearly forty unwanted pounds, into the lifestyle. They became my test subjects for all the recipe testing and food I prepared. At times I would lose their willingness to cooperate. I kept reminding them that we were still in the testing phase, and that one day I would make consistently delicious food that they would enjoy. Occasionally, they would try to get me to join them in returning to our old food, but after experiencing the incredible changes in myself, I had to firmly put my foot down and insist that we would never go back. I was feeling way too good with very little effort. In addition to the scientifically supported information that I was learning at the nutrition conferences, my extraordinary happiness, energy, and confidence inspired them, and gradually they began to buy in to this new way of life.

The deal was completely sealed for my husband after he saw one of the amazing studies in the documentary "The Game Changers," which extols the virtues of a plant-based lifestyle. After viewing he asked, "Where do I sign up?" The scene that grabbed his attention happens at the fifty-one-minute mark where the effects of a meat meal versus a plant meal are studied via the sleeping activities of Miami Dolphins football players. The findings in the film and at home were astonishing. The football players' reactions were priceless. My husband, who, with all the extra weight he had put on in middle age, had not been feeling as energetic as he once had, went on to tout the youthful changes he experienced with his friends. You will have to see the movie for yourself for further details as it is a bit embarrassing to discuss on a public platform, but let's just say he felt like a teenager again. The movie, narrated by WFPBD follower and bodybuilding great Arnold Schwarzenegger, is loaded with excellent information and will help you get a much better understanding of yourself and how simple it is to feel and look fantastic. Now, as I write this as the inhabitant of a healthy body, I am SO happy to have an opportunity to share with you the "secret" to reversing and avoiding disease that took me decades to learn and that has given my family a positive new life experience too. That brings me to why I wrote this book.

Why Eat Grass, Kick Ass?

When faced with the idea of a whole food plant-based diet, most people assume they must give up all the flavors they love, such as the taste of bacon, cheese, cookies, pepperoni, burgers, and seafood. I am here to tell you that that isn't true. Many people with allergies and other health conditions think they can't eat things they love on a WFPBD. Again, not true. *Anyone can make easy, delicious, homemade meals from whole food plant-based ingredients that will mimic their old favorite dishes, blow their minds, save them money, and change their lives in ways they could never imagine*—a fact that my family and I now know firsthand.

How did we switch to a WFPBD? you ask. Isn't it difficult? Won't it require eating lots of salad? Well, it really wasn't hard to do once we understood how a whole food plant-based diet really works and set some basic ground rules to follow. Let me also say that though this book is called *Eat Grass, Kick Ass: Plant-Based Done Right*, a WFPBD regimen is definitely NOT just about eating grass, so you don't have to fear that you'll only be eating salad for the rest of your life. My youngest daughter suggested the title, and, though I'm in the conservative profession of nursing and wondered if the name was a little risqué, I loved hearing people laugh wholeheartedly and express their admiration for the title when mentioned. I figured a moniker that could evoke a response like that would stick in people's minds and maybe have them come back for more . . . and change their lives for the better.

Who Needs This Book?

I wrote Eat Grass, Kick Ass, a combination nutrition-information and recipe starter book to help anyone who wants to live happier, healthier, longer, and to the fullest.

For people who eat pretty well already, such as vegetarians and vegans, the changes I recommend should be relatively easy to implement, and some positive changes will occur pretty quickly. For people who don't eat very well—think fried food, fast food, processed food, etc.—it may take a few weeks to become comfortable with this program, but you will likely see the most significant improvements of all. Your body will undergo positive physiological transformations. At the same time, your mind will undergo some psychological changes involving rewiring your perception of the food you've been programmed to eat all of your life.

To get to that point, you may need to remind yourself that plant-based eating will profoundly affect your health, appearance, feelings, and performance. Most of the time, the new food you will be trying will be heartier and more flavorful. At times, the textures may be more or less dense, but the flavors can be very similar to the food you already love.

Why This Book Is Special

Many books give you a general understanding of how plant food can reduce health problems, but they don't explain why it does and how to follow a WFPBD successfully. They don't show you how to give your favorite food a makeover by swapping in plant-based ingredients for the old, unhealthy ones. Eat Grass, Kick Ass, on the other hand, explains what a whole food plant-based lifestyle is, why it works, and how to make the food and recipes you already love healthier and tastier. It also provides excellent references, resources, and supporting evidence to prove how it can reduce and eliminate maladies, all of which can make this way of living last a lifetime. It shows you how this lifestyle can make you healthy and keep you that way.

In countless studies, the WFPBD has been proven to reduce or eliminate the top killers in our country: heart disease, cancer, and type 2 diabetes. It has also been proven to reduce or eliminate many other inflammatory diseases such as anxiety and depression, sleep disorders, joint pain, back pain, cramps, hot flashes, acne, and other skin disorders. It tends to make people feel light, energetic, happier, and younger. People find that they can reverse disease, reduce or eliminate their dependence on medications and other healthcare costs, and save a lot of money on food.

This Book Is Years in the Making

I have been a nurse for more than twenty years. I've cared for people in nearly every setting, from intensive care in open-heart surgery, neurology, and cancer to management of patients in home care and hospice. I've worked in communities and hospitals all over the country. Through rigorous nursing assessments and observations, and through discussions with patients and medical professionals, I have conducted my own personal research on the effect of food, not only on my family and me but on my patients' health as well. In so doing, I've seen the serious damage food can cause inside and outside of the human body. I've developed a strong belief that "food is thy medicine," and as a result, I have a passion for helping people establish healthy eating habits in order to extend and improve their lives.

As I was gaining nutrition knowledge over the years, I would refer patients to various sources to help them get on a path to healthier eating, but most of the sources were too difficult for the average nonmedical professional to navigate and understand. That's when I realized that all of this information, including the supporting research, needed to be pulled together and put it in one place—an easy-to-grasp book.

Today, however, more than just my patients want to know about a whole food plant-based way of life. They have spread the word about my experience with this lifestyle and people often approach me with questions about how to incorporate it into their lives. As my work continued on this book, I realized that I was writing it for all people, not just those with special conditions.

How This Book Can Help You

The primary purpose of this book is to eliminate confusion about healthy eating and to show you how to take control of your own health to achieve the highest level of wellness and happiness. Why do I feel a need to eliminate confusion?

Many times over the years, my attempts to provide evidence-based nutrition information have been met by pushback from those who get their knowledge from the Internet, TV ads, and other popular sources. Health magazine articles, hospital-provided teaching material, and even medical associations have caused confusion too. For example, in the hospitals many well-informed patients have asked me why their doctors advise them to eat one thing while nutritionists advise them to eat another. As a nurse, I have often shared my patients' frustration with this information disconnect over the years.

The truth is that the nutritional science research community, the food industry, the government, and educational institutions frequently put out conflicting information. But over the course of my own nutrition research, the incredibly informative nutrition conferences I have attended have provided clarity on key nutrition questions. The conferences led me to discover the work of a dedicated group of scientists who have been directly involved for many decades in nutritional scientific research studies. These scientists have not only been at the root of discovery and development of nutritional data, but they all support a whole food plant-based diet, primarily from organic or naturally grown sources rather than from synthetic or genetically modified sources.

Much of this book is based on their research. That said, *Eat Grass, Kick Ass* aims to clear up your own nutrition confusion and get you on the road to healthy eating in four parts:

* The first part of the book strives to help you decipher the facts from the Internet world of nutrition confusion by presenting scientific evidence-based information that will help you understand why a whole food plant-based diet is critical to helping you be healthy.

* The second part examines why there is so much nutrition confusion and which medical professionals are at the top in plant-based diet research, providing you information about their research and where to find more information.

* The third part looks at the impact of a WFPBD on specific populations, including pregnant women, children, and those with conditions including, but not limited to, cancer, celiac disease, gluten sensitivities, and allergies.

* The fourth part provides you with tasty meal alternatives and the guidance to help you create amazing plant-based replacements for the food you, your family, and your friends currently enjoy.

* The final flourish is recipes to help get you started with your new way of eating and a new lease on life.

Pay special attention to and explore the videos and websites referenced in this book as you will find that they are a treasure trove of great information that will open your eyes in ways you can't even imagine.

Expect Amazing Results!

Nearly everyone I know who has tried the program outlined in this book has experienced incredible health results and sticks to many features of a WFPBD, especially when they have access to proper resources, some guidance, and the information.

So let's start helping you prepare to embrace a better way of living. I'm about to guide you through the WFPBD lifestyle and clear up your nutrition confusion so that you'll become a health victor too. Let's help you do that by turning the page . . .

PART 1

Understanding A
Whole Food Plant-Based Diet

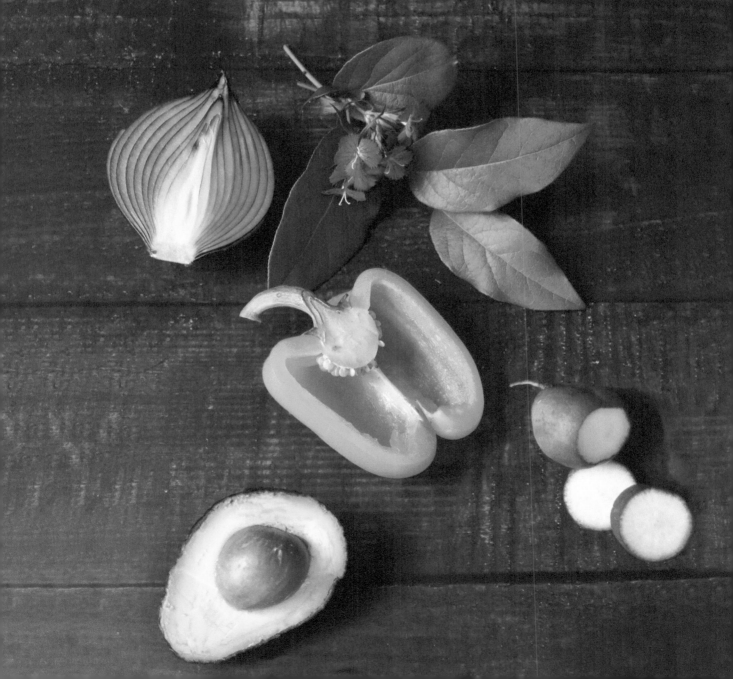

Chapter 1

We Need to Change What We Eat:
It's A Matter of Life, Disability, and Death

The State of Health in America

Before we jump into the basics of the whole food plant-based way of eating and wonderful recipes, we must take a deeper look into why we need to switch to this way of life. It's truly a question of quality of life and death, and it starts with the Standard American Diet, which is truly SAD as its acronym implies.

In hospitals, I have seen the result of people eating the typical American diet— excessive meat, poultry, eggs, dairy, and processed food that is packed with far too much protein, sugar, salt, fat, and many added cancer-causing chemicals. I've witnessed patients undergo cardiac catheterization for balloon angioplasties, a procedure where a stent is placed with a balloon expanded inside the heart vessels to open up the fatty vessel lining to increase blood flow. I've seen others undergo a procedure we sometimes call "roto-rooter" in which a surgical tool is spun inside the vessels to dissolve plaque. Cardiac procedures like these are high risk as one of the complications is that parts of a clot can break off and lodge in the brain, heart, or lungs, causing a stroke, heart attack, and even death. So, while that big juicy cheeseburger may look good to you now, what you should really be thinking about is not how it makes your mouth and mind happy for the moment but how it may seriously harm your entire body later.

Unfortunately, because so many of us Americans eat the SAD way, our health is considered among the worst in the world. Countless studies and statistics support this belief. Our country pays more per person than any other industrialized country for healthcare, yet we—as patients, undergoing heart surgery exemplify—are sicker.

Currently, our health with regard to obesity, heart disease, cancer, diabetes, and many other maladies continues to worsen. This puts us at great risk, especially when deadly viral diseases sweep through. Look at the 2020 COVID-19 pandemic with the increased morbidity rate among COVID-19 patients with pre-existing conditions. Most of the diseases that plague Americans are interrelated chronic inflammatory diseases that evolve into comorbidities or a collective group of disease that include conditions such as heart disease, obesity, diabetes, asthma, lower extremity edema, and more.

According to the National Center for Health Statistics at the Centers for Disease Control and Prevention, the biggest health crisis and number one killer in the United States, affecting a large portion of the US population is heart disease—the same disease that has afflicted my family members, who ate plenty of vegetables and fruit from our gardens but unwittingly continued to eat animal products, which contributed to their conditions. This silent killer that has plagued them currently slays about 647,000 Americans each year. More than 40 percent of Americans are obese, a contributing factor of heart disease, and more than 50 percent of them are taking prescription drugs, one of which is a statin drug for lowering cholesterol, and one of the most prescribed cholesterol-lowering drugs in the world[2]. Statin medications have several side effects, especially with long-term use. Myalgia, or muscle pain is the most common adverse effect, and rhabdomyolysis, resulting in kidney failure, sepsis, and death, is the most serious adverse effect. Other common risk factors include memory loss, confusion, sleeplessness, joint pain, hypothyroidism, multiple drug interactions, alcohol abuse, liver function complications, and the potential for the development of diabetes[3] and cancer. You can see why many people choose natural whole food remedies instead of statin medication for lowering cholesterol levels. Another common medication that frequently becomes a permanent part of ones life after a heart attack, arrhythmia develpment, or a catheter stent placment procedure are blood thinners. They are used to help prevent atheroclerotic fatty vessel disease, clotting, and help maintain stents that are placed for pressing open clogged vessels. Blood thinners require regular testing, monitoring, and adjustments to prevent reclogging and come with dangerous side effects including the risk of bleeding and stroke.

Cancer, the second leading cause of death in America, kills about 600,000 Americans per year. The total cost of cancer care continues to rise and is approximately 174 billion dollars annually.

Diabetes, another American health crisis, is consistently on the rise. In 2018, the American Diabetes Association reported that more than 34 million Americans had the disease, and almost 40 percent of deaths that occur in our country from multiple causes may be directly related to it but are undocumented or undiagnosed. In 2015, over 88 million Americans were prediabetic and about 210,000 Americans under age twenty were diagnosed with the disease. In 2017, the total cost of diagnosed diabetes was over 327 billion dollars. Our healthcare system is already overwhelmed and projections show a worsening trend and strain on our healthcare system.

Fortunately, the public is now beginning to understand that whole food plant-based diets can reduce or eliminate these diseases in our country. *We are beginning to understand that our overall health is a direct result of what we put into our mouths.* But more of us need to make the leap to understand this and to take action on our knowledge by adopting a whole food plant-based way of life.

We Don't Have to Be Sick

Genetics do play a role in whether we have a predisposition for certain diseases, but we have a tremendous amount of control over whether these genes are turned on or turned off. This has been shown repeatedly through careful studies on populations with shared cultural eating patterns and on families where people share the same genetic makeup, specifically identical twins. What they eat has clearly been demonstrated to determine whether they develop a particular disease or not.

Here's the crazy thing—as nutrition expert Dr. Michael Klaper has pointed out—if you talk to medical professors or open medical textbooks looking for the cause of many of these diseases or conditions, you'll often find these words: "Etiology (cause) Unknown." This prompts most doctors to prescribe medications to treat the symptoms, not the cause. The following is a list of inflammatory diseases which are caused by food. Scientists refer to this process whereby what we eat turns on and off genes as Nutrigenomics.

* Heart Disease (coronary artery disease, hypertension, angina, hyperlipidemia, hypercholesterolemia, congestive heart disease)
* Many Forms and Stages of Cancer
* Strokes (more than 90% of them)
* Obesity
* Type 2 Diabetes
* Peripheral Artery Disease
* Complications of Type 1 Diabetes
* Asthma
* Chronic Obstructive Pulmonary Disease (COPD)
* Allergies
* Metabolic Syndrome
* Crohn's Disease and Colitis
* Irritable Bowel Disease

* Constipation
* Chronic Kidney disease
* Reflux Disease
* Inflammatory Joint Pain
* Auto-immune Disorders
* Back Pain
* Arthritis Pain
* Cramps and Hot Flashes
* Impotence
* Infertility
* Acne and Itchy Skin Disorders Such as Psoriasis and Eczema
* Anxiety and Depression
* Dementia
* Unhealthy Weight Loss
* Sleep Disorders
* And Many Others

The fact is, most of these disorders, diseases, and conditions are curable. The hundreds of doctors who implement a lifestyle of nutrition as medicine have thousands of extremely happy patients who can attest to this fact and endless inspiring testimonials all over the world can easily be found. It disheartens me to know that the majority of Americans believe and anticipate that their health will naturally worsen in midlife, requiring them to take medications from that point on for the rest of their lives. It doesn't have to be that way. Though signs of health deterioration become evident in middle age, many studies and autopsies have clearly shown that heart disease, diabetes, and several other diseases actually begin in childhood, possibly even before birth. Fortunately, an abundance of evidence shows that diet can reverse many of these conditions and remove our need for dependence on medications and medical intervention.

It all comes down to "beefing" up the amount of vegetables, fruit, nuts, seeds, and grains we eat and eliminating or seriously minimizing meat, dairy products, eggs, salt, oil, and sugar.

How Dairy Products, Meat, and Eggs Harm Your Health

Studies show the dangers of animal sources of food in the Standard American Diet and its effect on our children, causing fatty vessel streaks in nearly 100 percent of them by the age of ten. Studies and health trends also show that the SAD has caused diabetes rates to soar. Dairy milk is a big contributor. As for meat, its protein level is too high for our digestive system to process and it does not contain two essential health-promoting factors-phytonutrients and complex carbohydrates containing fiber. Dietary fiber is comprised of soluble and insoluble parts. The soluble portion contains nutrients and the insoluble fiber is necessary to clear cholesterol from our complex, striated intestinal system. We store the extra protein and fat in our body tissues, organs, and vessels, clogging our hearts, brains, and cells.

As for eggs, according to Erin L. Richman et al., in study analyses published in The American Journal of Clinical Nutrition, it was shown that "men who consumed two and a half or more eggs per week had an 81% increased risk of lethal prostate cancer"[4] and in further studies, women who ate only half an egg increased their risk of breast cancer threefold. And no, only consuming the egg white and not the yolk is not a healthy alternative.

Why? you ask.

Nearly 90 percent of an egg-white is water, and while it doesn't have cholesterol, what it does have is a protein called avidin. One of the things avidin does is block our ability to absorb biotin, an important B vitamin that helps prevent hair thinning, skin rashes, fatigue, and depression. Additionally, when egg whites are heated, amino acids (more on these components of protein later) are damaged and form compounds that have been linked to various cancers and degenerative diseases. This damaged protein in cooked eggs also leads to the formation of end products known to accelerate aging.

Eggs, dairy, and meat, including fish and poultry, also cause our bodies to produce high levels of Insulin-like Growth Factor (IGF-1) and have been clearly shown to increase the risk of breast, prostate, colorectal, and lung cancer. IGF-1 is essential during development, but as adults, when the levels of IGF-1 remain high in our bodies, cells continue to multiply and develop into a variety of cancers and cancerous tumors.

A culprit that links all these different types of cancer-causing food is animal-sourced choline, an essential amino acid that our bodies don't produce. Choline from animal sources increases cancer risk by its involvement in producing a toxic compound called TMAO (trimethylamine n-oxide) in our gut—a substance that injures our vessel linings making vessel walls porous, creates inflammation, facilitates the formation of cholesterol plaques, and allows other toxins into our vessel walls[5, 6]—setting off a cascade of inflammatory diseases. Choline is so concentrated in cancer cells that if you follow it in the body, you can track the spread of cancer. The highest concentrations of animal sourced choline is found in eggs, but it is also found in milk, cheese, and meat, including poultry and fish.

Consider this: The New England Journal of Medicine reported the Cleveland Clinic research team's initial studies which showed that carnitine in steak caused spikes in the production of toxic TMAO. Carnitine is an amino acid that our bodies naturally produce and use to process fat and produce energy. The researchers decided to feed people hard-boiled eggs instead of steaks, and, just as they suspected, those who ate the eggs experienced a similar spike in TMAO as those who ate steak.[5, 6]. This shows us that not only do red meat and saturated fat play a role in causing heart disease and cancer, but that eggs, as well as meat and dairy, increase our risk of these diseases and many other inflammatory diseases regardless of our cholesterol levels because of their choline and carnitine content.

Fortunately, it appears as though the marketing and farming industries are beginning to demonstrate their understanding that animal products may not be the best food sources for us, and it is clearly evident that choline from plant sources like fruits, vegetables, whole grains, and nuts actually have healing effects. It's expected that commercials and marketing will lean far away from dairy milk in the near future, and many American farmers are transitioning to producing plant-based milk products containing soy, beans, grains, and nuts that include choline. New regulations have been set to limit and decrease commercialized animal processing[2], and I wouldn't be surprised if, in the future, a very high tax will be placed on those products as exists on tobacco and alcohol.

HEALTH IMPLICATIONS OF ANIMAL- AND WHOLE FOOD PLANT-BASED DIETS

These days, people are discovering that many delicious, high-quality *nonanimal* protein options meet and exceed expectations for helping them get healthy and lose weight. However, to understand the positive effects of a plant-based diet—newfound youth, energy, healing, weight loss, and so much more—you need to understand the impact of a diet that *includes animal* protein.

IGF-1 (Insulinlike Growth Factor 1) and Cancer

When we ingest animal protein, our bodies produce higher levels of the hormone IGF-1. This hormone is prominent during childhood and adolescence and levels off as we develop. It is involved in the growth of bones and muscles, and it helps manage and maintain blood sugar levels. Overproduction of IGF-1 in response to animal proteins is associated with a variety of common cancers in adults and children. It has been consistently associated with increased cancer risk, cancer cell growth, and malignancy[7, 8]. Animal proteins significantly boost IGF-1 production from our liver. The opposite happens in just a few days on a healthy plant-based diet, as IGF-1 levels drop significantly. Studies have shown that they can be lowered enough to reverse cancer growth in many situations. *Plant proteins reprogram the human body to slow down IGF-1 production, and animal proteins send a different signal to the liver to increase production.* Children with cancer have four times the levels of IGF-1 in their bloodstreams. However, you will not see the same type of damage with plant sources—that is, damage that can lead to the most common diseases in the US—and you typically cannot overdo plant protein.

Cholesterol, Carnitine, and Choline

Our bodies make all the cholesterol they need from the naturally balanced forms provided by plants, but extra cholesterol from animal sources lingers in the bloodstream, travels to the colon, and plays a significant role in many types of cancer. It also enters the lining of our arteries, cells, and other tissues after carnitine and choline enter our gut microbiomes, forming many compounds, including TMAO. Consuming cholesterol is problematic for human health because it increases our risk of developing heart disease, the number one cause of death for both men and women in the United States[2, 9, 10]. Undoubtedly, you already know that most animal food contains saturated fat and cholesterol. This is true for even "lean" meat such as chicken, turkey, and salmon, regardless of how it is grown, cooked, or prepared.

We've all heard the stories about marathoners and other athletes in seemingly great shape who unexpectedly and suddenly have a heart attack. This happens far more often than people realize. Many of these victims have a family history of heart disease and believe they can counter the possibility of ever having a heart attack simply by exercising and eating better than their parents. But a strong genetic cholesterol-elevating disorder can lurk in their bodies and hit them when they least expect it. Consuming animal protein and fat exacerbates this condition.

When working as a nurse in the emergency department, I clearly recall a very healthy-looking, lean man in his early sixties with impressive "collateral vessel mapping" that appeared on a scan of his heart. Everyone in the ER that day had never seen anything quite like it. Collateral vessels are small vessels that form to oxygenate the heart in response to narrowed coronary arteries due to atherosclerosis (fatty cholesterol build up in the arteries). They develop in people who continue to exercise, but they can only grow so far and support the heart for so long. This particular patient was one of those marathoners who ended up in the ER even though he thought he was doing everything he could to stay healthy. His family reported that he consumed a "regular healthy diet," which included lean, low-fat animal products.

This marathoner's story shows that genetics can play a strong role in this disease, but, again, even stronger is what you put in your mouth. I will say it again: *Our bodies make all the cholesterol they need, and any additional consumed cholesterol from animal sources is overkill . . . literally.*

Fortunately, countless heart attack patients have turned their health outlook around through diet conversion. I have encountered many of them as guest speakers at Dr. Dean Ornish's Lifestyle Medicine conferences. Many others speak at various health venues around the world. Their stories about how they transformed their lives and now show others how to do the same are incredible, heartwarming, and inspirational.

At a relatively recent conference, a speaker from my hometown of Virginia Beach told his story about his family history of heart problems. He said he was determined not to end up like his father, but one day on the treadmill at the gym, he suddenly dropped to the floor. CPR was performed on him, and he was rushed to the hospital. He was "dead" for eight minutes, at which point people commonly experience permanent brain damage and cardiac tissue death. Thankfully, he survived. He was referred to Dr. Ornish's program, which included stress management and changes in the way he was eating. He fully recovered, eliminated his elevated cholesterol level, which was 325 at the time of his heart attack—well above the threshold of 200—and signed a new lease on life. He now does motivational speaking engagements, sharing his remarkable story to inspire others.

NOTE: Meat does not contain any fiber, a critical cholesterol fighter—none, zero, zip. Yet it is commonly recommended as the "best source of complete protein." But it isn't, especially for those trying to reverse disease and eliminate the need for medications. Plants, on the other hand, have the highest fiber content. The only protein that has been proven, without a doubt, to reduce or eliminate disease, cholesterol, and weight is produced by plants. Only plants are loaded with antioxidants, complex carbohydrates, phytonutrients, and fiber. Fiber not only removes cholesterol from the body, lowering the risk of heart disease, but it has also been shown to help reduce the risk of stroke. Additionally, it is associated with decreased cancer risk, specifically colon and breast cancer, and lessens the risk of ulcerative colitis, Crohn's disease, constipation, diverticulitis, and high cholesterol[11]. If you are a typical American on the SAD, your fiber intake is less than half of the dietary recommendation[8]. No wonder heart disease is the leading cause of death in the US.

WAY BACK WHEN ... BEFORE FAST FOOD, PROCESSED FOOD, AND FACTORY-PROCESSED MEAT

Before World War II, the food available to the public was very different from today. Many of you have heard stories from your parents, grandparents, or great grandparents about how they all ate healthy garden vegetables and homemade food such as soups, stews, and bread. Typically, people rarely ate meat, and when they did, it was usually on Sundays and holidays, that is, if the family's hunter-gatherer was able to bring it home from the forest, marshes, plains, or a small and limited farm. Just prior to WWII, industries began to build equipment for increased animal processing, and focused on increased growth and production of animals for meat and milk supply. Many people also grew and ground their own flour from farm-grown whole wheat, whole rice, and oats. During the war, the healthy parts of the grains containing the nutrients were removed, leaving only the white starchy part, which was ground into white flour. This was done to increase shelf life and prevent bacterial growth so it could be shipped, stored, and fed to our soldiers overseas. During this time, the rest of the world became hooked on white flour too. Without the nutrients naturally found in the whole grains, the soldiers and many others around the globe developed diseases like pellagra and beriberi. The severe consequences of this white starchy food forced the industry to add back some of the nutrients, but many other more discreet diseases including ones previously mentioned in the group of interrelated inflammatory diseases remain in those who continue to consume it today.

During the war, a shocking thing occurred. Clear proof of the difference between eating meat or the alternative of living without it showed interesting results related to the impact animal food had on human health.

Fascinating studies and research evaluated and documented by Dr. Caldwell Esselstyn, Jr. on cholesterol, heart disease, and food consumption in Norway leading up to, during, and after the war support this amazing observation. The studies show dramatic changes when the Germans came during World War II and took away the livestock to feed their own soldiers. Heart disease dropped to nearly zero for Norwegians. When the livestock was returned, heart disease returned to dramatically high levels again. This is incredible evidence about the link between animal sources of food and heart disease.

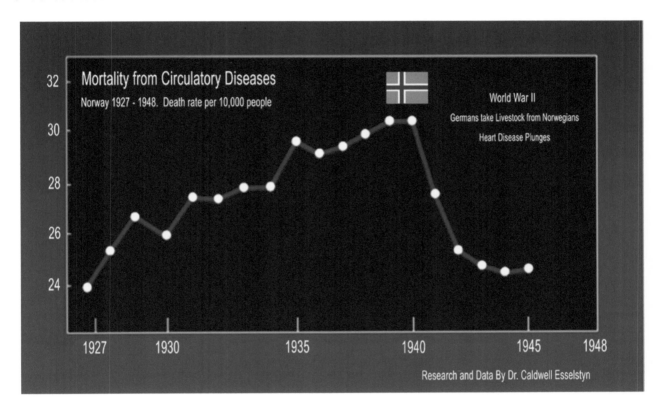

The food made available to Americans back then has undergone profound changes resulting in continuous and alarming disease trends. The development of processed food made with white flour, powdered eggs, and powdered milk, like boxed cake mixes, cookie mixes, and chips, has severely impacted our health. And food loaded with chemicals and preservatives like microwaveable TV dinners, bagged popcorn, and instant soup, have adversely affected our health. An examination of the health trends clearly shows vast increases in disease rates and the medications prescribed to treat them.

More Proof: The Blue Zones

"Blue Zones" are those few areas in the world where the healthiest and longest-living people over a hundred years old live with the highest-level quality of life, with little to no physical or mental limitations or disease compared to the rest of the world. That said, Loma Linda, California, is known as one of the world's Blue Zones. It consists mostly of Seventh-day Adventists. It is the only supercentennial community in our country, which means it has one of the longest living happy populations with the most 115-plus-year-olds. The inhabitants' longevity is attributed to several main characteristics, including regular exercise, a plant-based diet, family, social and spirituality engagement, stress reduction, avoiding tobacco, alcohol, and caffeine, and maintaining a healthy weight, all which comes easily on a plant-based diet.

With my own eyes, I've seen how people in the Blue Zones beat the American longevity odds. Nearly twenty years ago, when I worked as a nurse for Adventist Home Health and Hospice Care in California, I witnessed how differently Seventh-day Adventist patients handled recovering from surgery and how, at the end of their lives, they were generally older than most other hospice patients I encountered. It became apparent to me that their diet played a key role in their success. With my interest in health problems and eating patterns, I particularly remember many of these people in this small California town telling me that they were vegetarians or vegans. In the hospital, they would request salads without chicken or anything without meat, eggs, or dairy. This fascinated me, as it was common medical practice to encourage patients to increase their protein intake by eating sources from animals. I set out to learn more about their habits.

The Seventh-day Adventists traditionally eat two main meals per day: breakfast and lunch. Each community member may eat a little differently, but their food choices consist primarily of vegetables, fruit, whole grains, legumes (beans, peas, and lentils - some of the best plant-based sources of protein), nondairy products, and healthier fat such as that found in whole nuts and seeds. Most of them try to stay away from animal food, processed food, sugar, sugar substitutes, salt, and food additives. Studies performed on the Adventist Health communities with over 60,000 participants thirty years old and older showed that the more strict plant-based (or vegan) diet was associated with a body mass index (BMI) consistently lower than that of the vegetarians, pescatarians, ovo-vegetarians, and of course, the nonvegetarians[12]. Between their lower BMIs, overall better health, and increased longevity odds, the experience of people in the Blue Zones makes a strong case for the benefits of plant-based eating. The scientific community certainly supports the Seventh-day Adventists' way of life; and with the dedication of a rapidly expanding group of doctors and other medical professionals joining them to learn the principles of this diet and witnessing the miraculous improvements in thousands of lives, perhaps all of America will become a Blue Zone one day soon.

That is my fervent hope.

CHAPTER 2

What Is A Whole Food Plant-Based Diet?

Now that we've seen how a whole food plant-based diet can add happy, healthy, joyous years to your life, let's take a more in-depth look into what a WFPBD truly is by first looking at what it isn't.

The term "plant-based diet" first emerged in the health science community in 1980, specifically through the work of Dr. T. Colin Campbell, a biochemist who was researching at the National Institutes of Health, studying the effect of nutrition on long-term health. He wanted to distinguish between the impact of low-fat, high-fiber whole-vegetable-based food on cancer and to separate this type of diet from the terms "vegetarian" and "vegan."

Let's break these terms down to show some key differences between them and a whole-food plant-based diet:

Vegetarianism typically emphasizes consuming vegetables, fruit, nuts, seeds, and olive oil, but does not include meat though it often includes animal protein and cholesterol from eggs and dairy products. In contrast, whole food plant-based diets, include vegetables, fruit, nuts, and seeds, but also strongly emphasize whole grains and legumes (beans, peas, and lentils), including all parts of the food, hence making it "whole." The WFPBD ideally excludes meat, eggs, and dairy products entirely. Studies show that the microbiome (our digestive system) is able to safely clear TMAO with the seldom intake of very small amounts of animal protein in an otherwise strict plant-based diet regimen.

Veganism typically opposes raising and killing animals for food, based on concern for animals and the environment, and consequently often results in improved health for those who follow this way of eating compared to those who follow the Standard American Diet. A WFPBD, on the other hand, focuses on the nutritional impact of certain types of food on the individual person[13] rather than on ethical opposition to the killing or mistreatment of the animal.

Now, let's delve deeper into the history of the term "veganism" to show how it further differs from a WFPBD. The food industry treats these dietary approaches as being the same thing, but they aren't.

In the early 1900s, Americans primarily ate from their gardens and consumed minimal amounts of meat, traditionally on Sundays. Consuming farmer-raised chickens and cows was expensive and considered a luxury. After World War II, diets changed with the advent of fast food, TV dinners, boxed cake, cookie mixes, ice cream, and fried food. During this time, with the news of increased animal production and processing, the term "vegan" was coined to describe a diet free from all animal products.

In the past, vegans largely focused on avoiding animal products entirely for ethical reasons. This approach included any process that allowed plant food to touch animal products, such as when white sugar is filtered and bleached through animal bone char.

Today, the marketing industry labels processed vegan food as "plant-based" to take advantage of the public's heightened awareness of whole food plant-based diets. People often erroneously believe that "plant-based" and "vegan" are synonymous. Unlike whole plant-based food, however, vegan fare includes separated or isolated plant oil from olives, corn, avocado, safflower, coconuts, and sugar all of which can cause elevated cholesterol levels, weight gain, and cancer. It may also include isolated soy protein (ISP) and isolated gluten, aka vital wheat gluten, which is a suspect cause of imbalances resulting in gluten sensitivities, allergies, kidney damage, and cancer. A WFPBD, on the other hand, is void of these (we'll take a more in-depth look at ISP in Chapter 4).

Whole Food Plant-Based Diet Defined

The terms "*plant-based diet*" and "*whole food plant-based diet*" have been used interchangeably, but they are not the same either. That said, in this book, I'll use both terms to refer to the WFPBD to avoid having to repeatedly say "whole food plant-based diet," which can be a mouthful—no pun intended. Often, both terms basically mean the same thing to health-conscious individuals but adding the term "whole food" clarifies that you're eating food that has not been separated from its parts or in other words with no refined sugars, extracted oils, or isolated ingredients.

In 2013, with the clear recognition of the benefits of a WFPBD, *The New England Journal of Medicine* stated, "Healthy eating may be best achieved with a plant-based diet, which we define as a regimen that encourages whole, plant-based food and discourages meats, dairy products, and eggs, as well as all refined and processed food"[14].

The WFPBD Is Gaining Steam

As you may have seen in many grocery stores, demand has grown exponentially for organic nondairy milk and alternatives for everything, including butter, yogurt, cheese, and meat. The freight train of plant-based eating is here, and it is a new, and adventurous learning experience for everyone.

Grocery stores such as Whole Foods and Trader Joe's have some plant-based substitutes but navigating in stores to find them can be difficult. Over the next couple of years, these stores and others around the country are expected to increase the amount of whole plant-based food they offer, and it will behoove you to know more about them.

Some fast-food chains are carrying plant-based burgers and sausages. It can be a lot of fun to see the kinds of products that can be made primarily from plants but remember to use caution with these items as many of them contain isolated and chemically manufactured ingredients. (more on this later in the book).

Soy in its natural, whole food form is very beneficial, but overconsumption of soy protein in a concentrated form, as it is often found in many nonmeat fast-food burgers, appears to dramatically increase the production of IGF-1, the cancer-growth promoter mentioned in Chapter 1. Regular intake of any excess protein causes a lot of stress on the kidneys as they try to clear it from our bodies, and in worst-case scenarios, can lead to renal failure and the need for dialysis.

Producers of these products are being held more accountable by a better educated public and regulatory agencies. The expectation, supported by science, is that food selections will improve, and standards will continue to increase to safer levels. Stores are increasingly stocking organic ancient grains, beans, barley, whole grain chips, cookies, cereals, and varieties of previously unknown organically grown delicious vegetables like daikon root, jackfruit, hearts of palm, and baby bok choy. Organically grown produce typically contains 10-30% more nutrients than non-organic.

Healthy items unavailable in stores are easily found online. Online ingredients are often delivered within twenty-four hours. Sites like Amazon seems to carry everything the consumer needs, including more rare food, along with ratings and comments from customers.

A Few More Words about the WFPBD

Weight loss is the most significant change people notice after they immerse themselves in the WFPBD. Compared to other dietary approaches, the amount of weight one can potentially lose consuming only whole plant-based food is among the highest of all popular diets over a sixty-day period and the weight loss has been shown to last the longest. The math is easy. *There are four calories in one gram of complex carbohydrates (plants) and nine calories in one gram of saturated (animal) fat.* If you replace all fat with complex plant food, you could eat more than double what you normally eat, and the high-fiber content would likely fill you up first. Like thousands of others who have adopted a whole food plant-based diet, after you have converted your diet, you too will lose weight, feel great, and see your blood lab levels improve. The rewards are incredible, and you will ask yourself why you didn't know about this a long time ago.

As I know personally, having been a staunch consumer of whole plant-based food for years now, this lifestyle change can be easily maintained. Whole food plant-based eating is not a fad. Unlike other diets, once you've learned to adapt to it, it lasts a lifetime.

CHAPTER 3

The Basics: Setting Your Nutritional Foundation

In this chapter, I'll provide a short list of supplements to help you get off to a strong start as you begin a WFPBD. Once you've incorporated a variety of whole, healthy plant food into your eating regimen and get away from the SAD, taking some of the supplements on this list will become unnecessary. The rationale for this list appears on the pages that follow.

NOTE: The following suggestions are based on adult dose recommendations.

1. **Multivitamin:** daily, for those beginning a WFPBD and for those with poor diets. Not proven to benefit those eating a healthy WFPBD, though some experts continue to recommend multivitamins to cover all nutrient needs. Make sure whatever vitamins or supplements you take are from natural plant sources.

2. **B12, Cyanocobalamin**: daily or weekly, 50 micrograms (mcg) per day or at least 2,000 mcg per week while on any type of diet for life. Recommendations you see in most publicly accessible sources are much lower, but most nutritional scientists agree upon 50 mcg daily. B12 is considered a nontoxic, water-soluble vitamin, so there are no real concerns about getting higher than recommended amounts, because the body typically uses what it needs and disposes of the rest, but some doctors speculate that very high levels of B12 can interfere in metabolic processes in rare instances.

3. **Omega DHA/EPA:** daily supplement, 250 mg, and 1 tablespoon of flaxseed or 1-2 tablespoons of chia seeds, crushed and/or blended is recommended along with the best source of omega derived from algae to preserve and improve brain function, reduce heart disease, and extend longevity. Use these to replace dangerous forms of omegas (I will go into detail about this later in the chapter).

4. **Vitamin D3**: daily supplement, 2,000 IU (international units) is recommended unless you can acquire enough through your food and sunlight. Ideally, have your vitamin D levels checked and monitored.

5. **Iodine**: daily, 150 mcg. It can be covered in multivitamins, but ideally would be covered in a whole food plant-based diet.

Now, let's examine the items on this list.

Multivitamins

Multivitamins have not been proven to benefit people who consume a healthy diet and are certainly not as healthy as the plant food from which they are extracted or produced. In fact, scientific studies contradict one another about the benefits and risks of multivitamins and many indicate that multivitamins may not be necessary at all. However, taking a multivitamin may be a good idea if your dietary intake is questionable.

Other particular supplements are recommended that have been clearly proven to improve health in various ways no matter what type of diet you are on.

Note: For those who are pregnant, or could possibly become pregnant, consult with your obstetrician to determine prenatal vitamin and nutrient needs, as the baby's brain and heart development begin very early on, even before you know you are pregnant. Children should be seen regularly by their pediatrician and have dietary nutritional needs assessed and monitored while adjusting to a WFPBD.

B12: Cyanocobalamin

B12, cyanocobalamin is required for the proper function and development of the brain, nerves, blood cells, and many other body processes. It is crucial for preventing potentially irreversible neurological disorders.

It is not made by animals or plants. B12 is a natural vitamin produced from bacteria found in some soil, streams, and rivers. Humans used to get it from unwashed vegetables and from drinking from streams and rivers. Antibiotics and chlorine destroy it, and they also kill our natural intestinal bacteria designed to process B12. B12 can be consumed in food fortified with B12 like cereal, nondairy milk, and nutritional yeast, which is nutritious and rich in B12 and commonly used in plant-based food as a savory cheese flavor (check the nutrition label for B12 content).

More than 35 percent of the general population is deficient in B12, and that includes people who eat meat. The only part of the population that consistently has normal levels of B12 are those taking regular B12 supplements or those who are eating enough B12-fortified food. Most multivitamins contain about 4-6 mcg of B12. Most nutritional scientists recommend about 50 mcg per day or at least 2,000 mcg per week.

DHA/EPA . . . and ALA

Three types of omega-3 fatty acids are "essential" to the human body, meaning they must be acquired from our food. They are (alpha-linolenic acid) ALA, (eicosapentaenoic acid) EPA, and (docosahexaenoic acid) DHA. In their purest and healthiest form, all three of these fatty acids can be obtained from flaxseeds, chia seeds, walnuts, algae, and seaweed. ALA is the most common fatty acid found primarily in plant food and certain vitamins and minerals are required for converting it to DHA and EPA. Most people don't consume enough of the food containing these nutrients, so pre-formed supplements of DHA/EPA are recommended.

Omega-3 fatty acids are very important and have been shown to do many things in our body. They improve heart health by improving vessel dilation and blood flow which lowers blood pressure and reduces heart attack and stroke risk. They improve autoimmune conditions like rheumatoid arthritis by reducing overall inflammation, resulting in the reduction or elimination of associated joint pain. Omega fatty acids provide anti-aging effects resulting in healthier and younger looking skin and they help prevent dry eyes. They are beneficial for weight loss, decreasing asthma symptoms, reducing food allergy reactions, improving sleep, fighting depression, increasing the effectiveness of anticancer drugs and decreasing chemotherapy effects. They are essential for production of sperm and sperm health, with low intake of DHA as the most common cause of low-quality sperm and resultant infertility.

The DHA and EPA intake by pregnant women should be at a level to reduce the possibility of preterm birth, and in nursing mothers for proper development of their baby. Children also need adequate amounts of DHA and EPA, essential for brain and eye development, improving memory, learning, reducing impulsiveness, and increasing the ability to focus on tasks at hand. Interestingly, all of the things just noted are common symptoms of ADHD.

DHA comprises about 25 percent of the brain's total fat and enables nerve cells to send and receive electrical signals for mental processing. Our brains shrink as we age and by the time we are in our seventies, the average brain size reduces by about 26 percent. DHA and EPA are important for preventing brain shrinkage and may help prevent or slow Alzheimer's disease and other forms of dementia. Studies have shown that Alzheimer's patients have lower amounts of DHA and EPA in their brains than older adults with good brain function, and just after just six and a half months on supplementation, less brain shrinkage and significant improvement in executive function was noted.

Omega Sources to Avoid

In addition to DHA and EPA omega-3s, the fatty acid omega-6 from whole food sources also decreases inflammation, boosts brain function, and helps the immune system. When omega-6 is extracted and consumed as an oil, it is very dangerous. Sources of omega-6 oil are processed from safflower, sunflower, rapeseed (Canola), and cottonseed. These processed oils are typically made from genetically modified crops that are heavily treated with pesticides. To extract the oils from these plants, petroleum solvents and acids are used to remove the solids (the fiber and nutrients). Then it is heated and more chemicals are added to improve color and deodorize the oil. To make these oils solid for use as a margarine or spread, they are processed further through hydrogenation creating high concentrations of trans fatty acids or triglycerides which are known to increase total cholesterol levels and reduce HDL levels, making them one of the most dangerous forms of fat that cause heart disease.

Olive oil is not much better. Despite what you may have heard from many experts, olive oil is not a cure for heart disease. Monounsaturated oil extracted or processed from olives is stripped of its fiber and phytonutrients, disturbing the perfect balance of omega-3 to omega-6 fatty acids, causing inflammation throughout the body. Early studies were done to determine why Mediterranean diets were associated with lower heart disease and lower Alzheimer's rates. These studies mistakenly concluded that the olive oil provided the positive benefits they were seeing. As a result, people on a Standard American Diet increased their intake of olive oil. The result was that though HDL levels increased, total cholesterol levels did not decrease, nor did heart attack rates. Further studies showed that, while extra virgin olive oil retains some anti-inflammatory phytonutrients, it still significantly impairs endothelial function and is only slightly better than butter in this regard. More current expert opinion often dismisses olive oil as the explanation for the positive benefits instead. The higher intake of vegetables, including salads with whole olives, legumes, fruits, and nuts with balsamic vinegar in the Mediterranean diet, simultaneously with the lower intake of meat and dairy products is cited as the reason for the health benefits.

Fish and fish oil containing DHA and EPA have been touted throughout the Internet and other media sources as good solutions for eliminating heart disease and cancer. This has also been disproven with conclusive scientific studies showing that these sources have some serious cancer side effects, especially with regard to prostate cancer. Men with the highest blood levels of omega-3 fatty acids from fish were at the highest risk for this cancer. One of the persistent pollutants found worldwide in fish called PCBs (polychlorinated biphenyls) are also associated with a significant increased risk of stroke. A single serving of fish per week increases your risk of hemorrhagic stroke[15-17] and salmon has been shown to have some of the highest levels, putting it at the top of the list as being one of the worst.

A persistent pollutant can remain in your body for decades or forever. Many pollutants and contaminants are not only found in fish, but also in fish oil supplements. The contaminants found in fish oil supplements can cause neurological damage including ALS (Amyotrophic Lateral Sclerosis), Parkinson's disease, and Alzheimer's Disease. More than 80% of fish oil labeled as "pure" has been tested and remains contaminated[18]. Though fish oil has been shown to have no benefit for preventing a variety of disease, whole plant sources of omega-3s from flaxseeds and chia seeds do[19, 20].

Omega Sources to Incorporate

As mentioned earlier some of the best sources of omega-3 fatty acids are flaxseeds, chia seeds, walnuts, algae, and seaweed. Good sources of omega-6 include Brazil nuts, durum wheat, whole-grains, flaxseeds, hemp seeds, sunflower seeds, sesame seeds, poppy seeds, pumpkin seeds, cashews, pecans, pine nuts, walnuts, and soybeans. As you see, omega-3s and omega-6 are both contained in flaxseeds and walnuts, and not surprisingly, these and the others mentioned above are the healthiest form of omegas for the human body.

Algae contains significant omega-3 fatty acids and is considered the best source of omega oil containing DHA and EPA. This shouldn't come as a surprise since fish and krill feed on them. Algae is a better source of omega-3 in several ways: You get the same amount of EPA and DHA as you would from fish without the risk of toxic contaminants. Algae is very rich in vitamins and minerals such as iron, calcium, magnesium, and B12 and is known for its use in heavy metal detoxification from body organs, HIV/AIDS improvement, and cancer prevention.

With many similar benefits as algae, seaweed, a type of macroalgae, is another plant-based or vegan source of DHA omega fatty acid, but the levels of omega fatty acids are not typically as reliable or as abundant as those found in algae because of its lower fat content. Seaweed is an excellent source of iodine, which helps prevent hypothyroidism, a thyroid condition characterized by the low production of thyroid hormones. Seaweed can be added to any food for a seafood flavor including soups, stews, and plant-based ceviche, scallops, and crabcakes (See recipes).

In summary, nuts, seeds, and sea vegetables contain plenty of omegas, but many people have difficulty eating enough varieties of them to cover their needs, so experts recommend algae-derived omega supplements in addition to flax or chia seeds. As we age, dosing recommendations increase from about 250 mg to 500 mg or more per day.

A Few Words about Calcium

Since we're on the subject of DHA/EPA, let's take a moment to look at calcium, which is necessary to help metabolize ALA, EPA, and DHA. Calcium is richest in sources from the earth. Cows don't make the calcium found in their milk. They get it from grass, which is chockful of calcium. Cow's milk has been shown to leach calcium from our bones and has been associated with diabetes, including type 1 diabetes. Skim milk has also been shown to have a strong association to hip fractures and higher cancer rates in women[21]. Because the general population of a typical American diet does not contain sufficient calcium, supplements have been added to cow's milk and orange juice in accordance with the US Recommended Daily Allowance (RDA). In recent years, calcium supplements have also been strongly associated with many complications, including heart attacks, strokes, and increased death rates. In the United Kingdom, they recommend 500 to 1000 mg per day, specifically from dietary sources for most people, rather than supplements. If your doctor is prescribing you calcium, contact him or her and see the research at NutritionFacts.org: *Are Calcium Supplements Safe?* and *The Risk and Benefits of Calcium Supplements.*

All that said, why would you want to get your calcium from cow milk or supplements? The answer is, you don't have to. Soy milk and many other types of nondairy milk typically have about 45 percent more calcium than dairy milk, so check the nutrition labels. Dietary calcium can also be acquired through adequate amounts of these vegetables:

* Dark, Leafy Greens Such as Kale, Bok Choy, and Collards (and grass if you wish, lol!)

* Seeds Such as Sesame, Chia, Sunflower, and Poppy

* Beans Such as Soybeans (Tempeh and Tofu)

* Broccoli

* Nut Butters Such as Tahini and Almond Butter

* Nut Milks

* Molasses

Vitamin D and Other Fat-soluble Vitamins

Vitamins A, D, E, and K are fat-soluble vitamins that can be stored in our fat cells for long periods. Excessive amounts are not easily cleared and can cause damage, especially in those with kidney and liver disease and in the elderly. Vitamin D helps the body absorb calcium and phosphorus and is necessary for building and maintaining healthy bones. It helps facilitate the immune system, regulate the neuromuscular system, prevents cancer, and plays a significant role in the life cycle of cells. The best vitamin D source for increased longevity and vitality is D3, which is the active form that is acquired from the sun, produced in our skin, and readily utilized. Vitamin D2 is usually obtained from plants like mushrooms but in varying levels and in nuts, seeds, shiitake, portobello, chanterelle mushrooms. It is also found in fortified food with vitamin D, such as nondairy milk, tofu, cereal, and orange juice. If you spend a lot of time indoors or often use sunscreen and do not take any supplements, you are likely low in vitamin D and should take a supplement of 2,000 IUs (International Units) per day. This is an especially important practice in the winter or if you live in zones where the sun is not as abundant.

Iodine

We need iodine for the production of thyroid hormones and thyroid function, energy conversion, and many other body processes. Pregnant women need iodine to control their blood pressure and prevent stunted growth and altered brain development of the fetus[22]. Most women don't get enough iodine during pregnancy, and only about half of prenatal multivitamins contain any iodine at all. The National Institutes of Health states that the RDA for US women who are pregnant, lactating, or even planning a pregnancy should be increased to 220 mcg of iodine per day and 290 mcg per day for breastfeeding[23]. During pregnancy, iodine is necessary for preventing stunted growth and altered brain development of the fetus[22]. See the excellent video *Supplements Before, During and After Pregnancy* at NutritionFacts.org.

Iodine deficiency can lead to an enlarged thyroid gland and autoimmune disease of the thyroid, which may increase the risk of thyroid other types of cancer. A deficiency may alter ovulation, leading to infertility. In the early 1900s, the US government realized that the severity of health consequences in certain northern and western US regions was related to low iodine. The soil in these regions contained little to no iodine. As a result, in 1924, salt companies added iodine to its salt at the government's request. This table salt came to be known as "iodized," and its consumption was encouraged to prevent related health complications. Iodine is an element we can acquire through food like potatoes, navy beans, black beans, grains, peas, cranberries, strawberries, corn, prunes, nuts, and nondairy milk which is often fortified with it. People typically don't consume enough of these to get enough iodine on a Standard American Diet.

Recently, iodine has again become a big concern, with people moving away from iodized table salt and consuming alternatives like kosher and sea salt, as they have only traces or complete absence of iodine. Most of the world's iodine is found in the ocean, concentrated in sea life, especially in seaweed. Certain seaweed has been shown as not only the best source for iodine but is also believed to prevent cancer and may have a therapeutic effect on people fighting liver cancer. Seaweed is full of vitamins and minerals, and the best sources of it come in convenient packaging to snack on. You don't need to eat much of it. You can eat it plain or mix it in your food by flaking it up in sandwiches or soup or consuming it in plant-based versions of sushi, crabcakes, and ceviche, just as you would to acquire healthy omegas. The recommended dose of iodine is 150 mcg per day. Varieties of seaweed like dulse, laver/nori, alaria, and wakame are the recommended sources. Kelp is another source that is very high in iodine, but it is not normally recommended unless you can limit kelp intake accordingly. Kelp powder or flakes are available, and a little can be added to a shaker of a salt substitute or other seasoning made from herbs and spices. Maine Coast Sea Vegetables is one of the producers found online for many sea vegetables.

As you have seen, certain supplements are still recommended no matter what type of diet you are on. As your practice of eating whole plant-based food improves and expands, you'll get the nutrients and vitamins required to meet all of your nutritional needs.

CHAPTER 4

The Protein Question Examined

When my patients, friends, and family began learning about plant-based diets, one of the first questions they asked is whether a plant-based diet provides enough protein. My answer is: "Absolutely! You get more than enough!" Their eyes light up with complete surprise. We've all been living in a world where this fact has long been an illogical fallacy.

The fact is, our bodies do not need as much protein as people think and you can easily meet all of your body's protein needs by eating plant-based food. Protein is readily available throughout the plant kingdom, and the food that is particularly rich in protein includes legumes, nuts, nut butter, seeds, seed butter, soy food, and whole grains[24]

Let's establish what protein is and does. Protein is critical because it is a component of every cell in the body. It repairs tissues, makes enzymes, makes hormones and builds bones, muscles, cartilage, skin, and blood. Protein ensures the proper functioning of the immune, circulatory/blood, digestive, and nervous systems. We need it for wound healing and maintaining a healthy weight. We need it for energy and to balance our body fluids to prevent edema/swelling.

Protein is made up of amino acids. There are twenty necessary amino acids required for our body to function properly. Our body can make eleven of these proteins, but the other nine must be acquired from our food, and they are called "Essential Amino Acids." To obtain all nine essential amino acids, we must consume a variety of food on a regular basis. There are some powerful healthy plant food sources like soybeans, flaxseeds, quinoa, and buckwheat that contain all nine of the essential amino acids plus some that our bodies make, but we still need a variety of food in our diet for many other health benefits. Let's take a closer look at each essential amino acid and reveal specific ways they help the human body.

THE ESSENTIAL AMINO ACIDS

What Are the Nine Essential Amino Acids?

The nine essential amino acids are histidine, isoleucine, lysine, leucine, methionine, phenylalanine, threonine, tryptophan, and valine. Some of the best sources of the essential amino acids come from the following: legumes such as chickpeas, soybeans, navy beans, black beans, kidney beans, peas, and lentils; whole grains such as buckwheat, oats, quinoa, brown rice, and rye; nuts such as peanuts, walnuts, cashews, almonds, Brazil nuts, hazelnuts, and pine nuts; seeds such as sunflower, hemp, pumpkin, sesame, chia, and flax; leafy greens such as kale, parsley, spinach, watercress, bok choy, and seagrasses/vegetables; vegetables such as white potatoes, broccoli, corn, eggplant, sweet potatoes, squash, zucchini, cauliflower, Brussel sprouts, asparagus, cabbage, winter squash, beets, corn, carrots, mushrooms, celery, carrots and pumpkin; and fruit such as guavas, avocados, jackfruit, raisins, dates, apricots, bananas, kiwi, blueberries, and cantaloupe.

Let's break down each of the nine essential amino acids:

* **Histidine** is involved in growth, the creation of blood cells, and tissue repair in the body. It is converted to histamine, which acts as a neurotransmitter for immune response, digestion, sexual function, and sleep-wake cycles. It maintains the protective barrier surrounding our nerve cells—the myelin sheath.

* **Isoleucine** is involved in wound healing, detoxification, stimulating immune function, blood sugar regulation, and hormone production. It's also essential for hemoglobin production (the oxygen-carrying protein of a blood cell), energy level regulation, and assisting in healing muscle tissue.

* **Leucine** produces growth hormones and helps with endurance and repair of muscle and bone. It also helps regulate blood sugar levels, stimulates wound healing, and helps reduce depression.

* **Lysine** builds muscle, aids in recovery from injury or surgery, and is involved in hormone and enzyme production and regulation, absorption of calcium, and strengthening bones. It's also vital for energy production, immune function, carnitine, collagen, and elastin, and preventing depression. It may also have antiviral effects.

* **Methionine** plays an essential role in metabolism and detoxification and is necessary for tissue growth. It aids in the absorption of selenium and zinc and removes heavy metals, such as lead and mercury. Methionine helps fight bacteria in urine, reduces edema, helps prevent arthritis, and plays a role in skin and hair's health and flexibility, and strengthening fingernails and toenails. It helps boost the mood-lifting hormone serotonin and improves the functional ability of people with Parkinson's.

* **Phenylalanine** is an essential amino acid involved in the structure and function of many proteins and enzymes. It is a catalyst for converting tyrosine and several neurotransmitters, including dopamine, epinephrine (adrenaline), norepinephrine, and the skin pigment melanin. Dopamine is involved in the feeling of pleasure in your brain, forming memories, and learning skills. Epinephrine and norepinephrine are integral components of the fight or flight response. Phenylalanine may help treat depression, pain, and Parkinson's disease symptoms.

* **Threonine** is necessary for healthy skin and connective tissue as it is an integral component of collagen and elastin. It also plays a role in fat metabolism, immune function, muscle repair, heart health, and liver health and may be beneficial for indigestion, anxiety, and mild depression. It is also a necessary component of tooth enamel.

* **Tryptophan** is necessary for maintaining proper nitrogen balance and muscle growth and is a precursor to serotonin, a neurotransmitter that regulates your appetite, sleep, and mood. Tryptophan may help improve mental energy and emotional processing.

* **Valine** is essential for muscle growth and coordination, tissue repair, energy production, mental focus, and emotional calm.

Complete Proteins

As previously mentioned, complete proteins are those that include the *nine essential amino acids* our bodies cannot make independently. The eleven amino acids our bodies do make on their own are called nonessential amino acids. Our bodies are naturally designed to combine the essential and nonessential amino acids to form proteins. Incorporating a variety of fruit, vegetables, legumes, nuts, seeds, and whole grains provides all the amino acids, protein, vitamins, and minerals we need. Plants are the best source of protein because they do not adversely affect our bodies and cause disease.

Complete proteins come naturally from a wide variety of plant-based food. The good thing is, you don't even have to think about them on a plant-based diet. It is not necessary to eat complete proteins with every meal because our bodies are smart enough to keep a supply of essential amino acids on hand for days to match up with the nonessential amino acids for the creation of complete proteins.

Food combinations that please our palate naturally happen to be complete proteins:

* Whole Grain Pitas or Chips with Hummus

* Peanut Butter on Whole Grain Bread

* Rice and Beans

* Bean Chili with Whole Grain Bread

* Whole Grain Noodles or Rice with Peanut Sauce or seeds

* Beans with Corn

* Whole Grains with Lentils

* Fruit Jam on Whole Grain Bread

* Peanut Butter and Banana

* and Many More

Examples of Complete Proteins

Examples of complete protein food include soybeans, tempeh, nutritional yeast, farro, flaxseeds, hempseeds, quinoa, amaranth, buckwheat, soba (buckwheat noodles), and chia seeds. Soy is a complete protein source and comes in the form of edamame (soybeans), tempeh (fermented soybeans), miso, tofu, and soy milk. Interestingly, tofu (made from soybeans) is partially processed and loses some of its nutrient content but is still rich in protein, retaining about 40% of its nutrient quality. Ezekiel bread, another complete protein, is made from sprouted grains, legumes, and pumpkin seeds. This bread reduces the risk of heart disease and stroke, improves blood sugars, boosts mood, helps with sleep, boosts the immune system, supports bone health, and helps with collagen and elastin production, cellular repair, and overall anti-inflammatory processes. Eating a variety of plant-based protein throughout the day provides the body with a complete amino acid pool from which it can make protein for all body functions and processes. It is easy to meet and even exceed protein requirements without even thinking about it once proteins are understood.

Adequate intake of protein is based on recommended/expected ideal weight and is estimated as follows:

Age Range	Infants	1 to 3 years of age	4 to 13 years of age	14 to 18 years of age	Adults	Pregnant and lactating
Recommended Protein in grams/kg/day	1.5	1.1	0.95	0.85	0.8	1.1

To calculate recommendations of protein for the average 150-pound adult: 150 divided by 2.2 (kg) x 0.8 = 54.5, rounds to *55 grams* of protein per day. And for the average 90-pound child, *39 grams* of protein per day is recommended. Any more than that, as noted earlier is overkill and can cause disease, early disability, and death. An 8 oz steak contains about 37 grams of protein and a quarter pound cheeseburger contains about 33 grams protein. As you will see below, this amount of protein is easily met in one plant-based meal (dinner) containing nothing but healthy disease-reversing food without calculating in any other meal or snacks eaten in a day.

Many sources at your fingertips recommend calculating protein needs based on half of your body weight, but this method doesn't work very well for those who are overweight. Athletes will need to bump it up a bit, based on the additional protein used, but consuming too much of the wrong type of protein can seriously damage the kidneys, among other things mentioned earlier.

Now, let's look at the total protein you can easily consume on any given day from a whole food plant-based diet. The chart that follows should make it easy to see that you don't have to count protein to easily meet your protein needs. It is not necessary to be concerned about what you're eating as long as you follow the basic rules of sticking to whole plant-based diet. The chart will show you sample meal ideas and protein totals.

Total Protein in an Average Whole Food Plant-Based Day

Selection	BREAKFAST OPTIONS			Protein in Grams
1	Whole grain bread, 2 slices (12)	1/2 Avocado w/ cilantro, onion, tomato (3)	Oat Milk, 1 cup (7)	22
2	Tofu scramble wrap (11)	2 slices tempeh bacon (8)	Orange, banana, and blueberries (2)	21
3	Whole grain cereal, 1 cup (10)	Soy milk, 1 cup (7)	Nuts, seeds, raisins, 1/4 cup (5)	22

Selection	LUNCH OPTIONS			Protein in Grams
1	Quinoa and lentil burger, 1 patty (12)	Whole grain bun (7)	Salad (2)	20
2	Beans, rice, and hummus burrito, 1 medium (9)	Bell peppers and Greens (2)	Whole wheat wrap (6)	17
3	Chickpea salad (6) [sandwich]	Whole grain bread, 2 slices [Dave's] Killer Bread (10)	Fruit and/or vegetables (2)	18

Selection	DINNER OPTIONS			Protein in Grams
1	Whole wheat spaghetti w/tempeh crumbles, 1 cup (22)	Green salad (2)	Whole grain garlic bread, 2 (12)	36
2	Quinoa, lentil burger (17)	Whole grain bun (7)	Baked beans, 1 cup (14)	38
3	Vegetable bean chili, 1 cup (20)	Veggie cheese, onion, cilantro toppings (2)	Whole grain dinner rolls, 2 (11)	33

Selection	SNACKS OR DESSERTS	Protein in Grams
1	Edamame, 2/3 cup	13
2	Hummus, 1/2 cup (11) and chips (2)	13
3	Chia pudding, 1/2 cup - soy milk (7) and 1 tbsp seeds (6)	13
4	Bean Dip, 1/2 cup (8), whole grain crackers (7), apple slices (2)	17

These meals are all based on single servings for the average person and, in most cases, determined by nutritional data labels. Many men will double their portions, and as you can see, it is effortless to get all the protein you need from a plant-based diet. To further help you determine what constitutes a single serving size, refer to the American Heart Association's recommendations below:

Grains: 1/2 cup cooked rice, pasta, or cooked cereal; 1-ounce dry pasta or rice; 1 slice bread; 1 cup ready-to-eat cereal flakes

Vegetables: 1 cup raw vegetable or vegetable juice, 2 cups leafy salad greens

Fruit: 1 cup equivalent is 1 cup fruit or 1/2 cup of pure fruit juice

Beans, Nuts, and Seeds: 1/4 cup cooked beans; 1 tbsp peanut butter; 1/2-ounce unsalted nuts/seeds

Milk and Yogurt: 1 cup milk or yogurt

Now that you've seen how easy it is to get your protein through plant-based food, let's look at one source to be cautious of - isolated soy protein.

Isolated Protein and "Plant-Based" Burgers

Isolated soy proteins (labeled ISP or SPI), or extracted plant proteins, as mentioned in Chapter 2, can be very harmful to the kidneys. ISPs are found in many "plant-based" or vegan burgers, hot dogs, luncheon meats, sausages, candy bars, shakes, and cheeses. Isolated soy proteins are deficient in natural dietary fiber or complex carbohydrates, vitamins, minerals, and phytonutrients. Food containing ISPs are currently very popular, but scientists are concerned about their implications for the public's future health. For those who think that ISP food is doing them good, consider that 40 grams of *isolated* soy protein increases the cancer growth promoter, IGF-1 by 69 percent, while whole soybeans have the opposite effect by reducing cancer. We already know that our genetics play a role in our risk of developing cancer and heart disease, but this concern applies even to those who don't have a family history of cancer.

People often ask which is worse; a cheeseburger made with meat or a "plant-based" burger. We already know that *plant-based* is not the same as *whole food* plant-based. Go to Dr. Campbell's site, NutritionStudies.org to compare the nutritional data at https://nutritionstudies.org/fake meats how do beyond and impossible burgers stack up from a health perspective? You will see that the popular "plant-based" burgers available today contain genetically modified ingredients, isolated proteins, high levels of processed oil, saturated fat, extremely high levels of sodium, starches, extracts, and chemicals. Both "plant-based" or in actuality, *processed burgers* and beef burgers promote cancer and a variety of inflammatory chronic diseases. Best advice is to minimize or avoid animal products and processed food. Instead, eat non-GMO, whole food sources made from plants with clean protein and phytonutrients like edamame, tofu, beans, lentils, nuts, seeds, and fermented sources like tempeh and miso *which actually reverse disease*.

Soy Is A Good Protein, Despite What People Say

People have been told that soy is an estrogen that causes breast and prostate cancer. It *is* a type of estrogen, but estrogen from soy is a plant source called phytoestrogen. It has the opposite effect of animal-based estrogen on humans. It competes with animal estrogen by blocking it from receptors, reducing breast and prostate cancer risk. Most of the confusion swirling around soy stems from the fact that the older studies were conducted on a different species, such as rodents. Years later, the opposite results were produced when the studies were performed on humans, but news and industry sources have been remiss in informing the public.

Studies showed many beneficial effects for women who consumed soy and soy's ability to fight cancer. Thousands of women in each study showed that when they ate soy, they lived longer, had lower cancer recurrence rates, and greater survivorship by about 30 to 40 percent[25-27].

Study reviews have led the FDA to conclude "that many soy products should be beneficial to cardiovascular and overall health because of soy's high content of polyunsaturated fats, fiber, vitamins, minerals, and low content of saturated fat." The FDA granted a health claim that "25 grams of soy per day should be part of a diet low in saturated fat and cholesterol and may reduce the risk of heart disease, and by replacing soy for many of the other harmful animal products, overall human health is much improved." The American Cancer Society concluded that soy is beneficial as well.

Soy has not only been proven to reduce heart disease and be a cancer fighter but to have numerous other health benefits too. For example, studies in Japan performed on women who had two bowls of miso soup, with a total of about 1/2-1 teaspoon of salt daily, depending on the amount and type of miso, showed a five times lower risk of hypertension (high blood pressure). The average American consumes about 3,400 mg of salt (sodium) per day, nearly 50% more than is generally recommended. More than half of Americans are hypertensive and more than 20% more are unaware that they are. It is believed that the soy in miso may be countering the harmful effects of the sodium[28, 29]. In the June 2003 issue of the Journal of the National Cancer Institute, studies showed that Japanese women who consumed two bowls of miso soup per day also had lower breast cancer rates and cardiovascular disease. Not that miso is recommended, necessarily, but simply pointing out the benefits of soy in general. Another example: hot flashes are prevalent in older women in America and Europe but are rare in Japan, where soy is frequently consumed. In 75 percent of studies, soy phytoestrogens have been shown to significantly reduce hot flashes. Women who consumed four ounces of tofu per day cut their hot flash risk in half compared to those who ate one ounce per day[30]. Tofu is the curd from soybeans and has a lesser amount of soy. Studies have shown that estrogen pills also reduce hot flashes, muscle pain, joint pain, and dryness. The estrogen pills have been proven to be somewhat more effective than soy, but soy phytoestrogens are more highly recommended because they provide the benefits without the increased risk of breast cancer, uterine cancer, or cardiovascular disease that has been associated with estrogen pills. In addition to reducing menopausal and menstrual symptoms, soy is beneficial for bone density, preventing bone loss, bone fractures, and osteoarthritis.

A common concern among men in relation to soy is that the phytoestrogen in it would cause feminine or androgen effects. This is an unnecessary concern as research shows that a man would need to consume about five liters of soy milk per day to encounter any feminine effects. It's far more likely that the estrogen levels contained in beer hops would cause feminine characteristics in men than soy ever would[31]. See the video *Soy and Cancer* on NutritionFacts.org.

The Moral of This Story: Don't Be Afraid of Soy.

Meeting Protein Needs Is a Breeze

As the information in this chapter has demonstrated, eliminating all animal protein from your diet will not make you protein deficient. On the contrary, as your daily eating regimen begins to consist of a variety of whole plant-based food, you should be meeting your protein needs without any problem. Make this way of eating a way of life, and good nutrition will naturally fall into place.

CHAPTER 5

How to Begin a Whole Food Plant-Based Diet

Retrain and Redesign

CAUTIONARY NOTE: *Before Changing Your Diet, Notify Your Doctor If You Have Any Underlying Conditions.* If you are diabetic, tell your doctor that you are embarking on a whole food plant-based eating regimen and that you anticipate that your insulin medications will need to be reduced. Whole food sweeteners can dramatically decrease blood sugar levels because of their low glycemic index (a sugar spike indicator that ranks food based upon its effect on blood sugar levels). This new way of eating may mean that you can eventually eliminate medications altogether.

The first step to beginning a whole food plant-based diet is to be open to embracing it. This may seem like an obvious statement, but many people don't give the program the time and consideration needed to reach their nutritional goals.

I know this from my many years as a nurse.

While practicing nursing in hospitals, the most eye-opening experiences occurred when I assisted with surgical procedures called a carotid endarterectomy. During this procedure, fatty plaque is removed from the carotid arteries of the neck. This is significant as these are the arteries that provide blood flow to the brain. I was able to see first-hand how fat can clog and solidify within our vessels. Doctors routinely pull fatty plaque that looked like large round French fries out of patients' neck vessels. Some of these fatty plaque strips contained tiny tunnels where blood could barely flow through to the brain. The fortunate patients were those who had this procedure done before permanent damage was done to their brain. Following this procedure and others like the ones mentioned earlier (balloon angioplasties and "roto-rooter"), patients would share their excitement about how they no longer felt dizzy, were no longer experiencing chest pain, and loved the sensation of the increased blood flow to their legs, which was enabling them to walk again. They spoke about how they experienced improved breathing, restored energy, endurance, and so on. Sadly, we often knew their after-surgery gains would be temporary as we would see many of them repeatedly. These patients were what we called "frequent flyers" because they returned repeatedly. Why? Because though they would go out the door with every intention to change their eating habits and improve their lifestyle, they would often fail. For that I blame the enormous disconnected system and all the insdustry and media-propagated confusion.

It always surprised me how some people, after having undergone significant procedures like open-heart surgeries, amputations from diabetes complications, or a lung resection from cancer, would ask their families to bring them pizza, burgers, soda, candy, fries, or cigarettes, as if going through the surgery or recovering and graduating from the ICU made them deserve a reward like that. Family members and friends would walk right in, serve up the offerings, and eat it with my patients. Patients would beg to be allowed to go outside for a smoke, even after they made a pact with their surgeons prior to surgery that they would quit smoking permanently. Many surgeons refuse to operate on these patients unless they agreed to this pact. Patients didn't understand that we had just spent our entire fourteen-hour+ shifts doing all we could to keep them alive only to see them repeat habits that led them to be our patient in the first place. It would make me want to throw my hands up in the air and cry.

These patients are not necessarily the minority. Many of us have lifelong bad habits that they do not recognize as problematic. These habits make them more dependent on the medical system with frequent doctor appointments, medications, surgeries, and multiple procedures. They could potentially have a way out if they just gave change a serious try. A Whole Food Plant-Based Diet would be a solution. If the individual patient could find a way to focus on how much it can improve their health, appearance, and general overall feeling as they go through the process, they might actually find health success. Most people who do succeed agree now that no amount of pizza, burgers, or fries made with animal products is worth shaving happy, healthy years off your life. A WFPBD can change your life for the better *for the rest of your life*. So, let's look at how to begin your new lifestyle. Let's get ready to embrace it! This starts with retraining your taste buds.

Retrain Your Taste Buds and Redesign Your Microbiome (Your Gut)

Our microbiome consists of over 39 trillion microorganisms, all living in either chaos or perfect harmony based on what we eat. From the beginning, our bodies have the potential for craving healthy selections of food. Humans are naturally driven to eat high-calorie food. You would think that infants would select sweet food over anything else, but many studies show that they tend to pick healthy fare that is naturally high in calories and nutrients. Many children brought up on plant-based diets continue this selection process and reject lower-calorie, nonnutritional food. For example, whole grains have high-caloric density, but when children eat unnatural, processed food with high calories—like cheese, sugar, white bread, and candy—they tend to forget about the healthy high-calorie food and select the food chemically designed to capture their attention instead. When our brains' pleasure systems are activated, and the hormones are released to identify and remember things that make the brain happy (not necessarily healthy), the same area of the brain that opioids or narcotics activate is turned on. Once we are exposed to it, our brains have a lot of difficulty forgetting about it, and it becomes an addiction[32].

As a nurse, I have helped people who are addicted—mostly to cigarettes, but also to drugs, alcohol, and unhealthy food. I would teach these individuals to understand the core urges of their addiction, the changes that take place in the brain regarding receptors, pleasure center activity, dopamine, and the damage that brain-altering substances can cause. Some of this damage includes memory loss, Alzheimer's, heart disease, premature aging, and of course cancer, heart, and lung disease. With a lot of determination and self-control, many can reverse damage and even quit smoking by staying focused on reaching a goal of six months of abstinence. We all know this is harder than it sounds but having a foreseeable and attainable goal seems to work well for most people. At each month mark, many patients have been thrilled to express their ability to avoid the triggers and the addiction source. And after six months, they have successfully managed to avoid reactivating the addiction forever. Food addictions work much the same way when you retrain your taste buds and redesign your microbiome with healthy microorganisms, but it is said to be much easier than stopping smoking.

Start out retraining your taste buds by cutting back, eliminating, or as most would say is even better....replacing sugar, oil, and salt with healthier alternatives. I'll be going into detail about this in upcoming chapters, but first, I want to share what I learned about some of the most popular unhealthy food during my many years of traveling around the world as a military spouse. My story will lay a foundation to help you prepare to retrain your taste buds to enjoy healthy food and change your life. For many of you, this information will be an eye-opener!

So You REALLY Think It's the Meat You Like? Think Again.

As I visited my husband in his various ports or met people from different countries during our travels, I became familiar with food flavors from around the world including places like Mexico, Thailand, England, Italy, Greece, and Canada. As time passed, it became clear that the distinct and delicious flavors were not the underlying food, necessarily, but the variety of herbs, spices, sauces, and vegetables they were prepared with. For instance, I discovered that the real flavor of sausage is the fennel, black pepper, garlic, and salt. I can't even imagine how bad pork scraps would taste without those seasonings. Unseasoned seafood actually tastes like the food the fish eat and drink—seaweed and sea salt. Seaweed by itself is quite healthy and has a salty ocean flavor, but add some seasonings like garlic, herbs, salt, or Old Bay and you have a tasty treat. Bacon is quite delicious because of the salt, smoke, pepper, and maple flavor. Poultry gets its flourish from the sage and salt. It's definitely the butter, salt, garlic, parmesan, and herbs with lobster and escargot. Mexican cuisine is all about cumin, chili powder, hot and sweet peppers, tomatoes, onions, cilantro, avocados, and Italian flavors are all about tomato, basil, fennel, olives, and oregano.

The moral of this tale? If you didn't load up these dishes with various herbs and spices and other enhancers, you probably wouldn't eat them. Use some of these same ingredients—the healthy ones—to transform your food to retrain your taste buds. This just requires some creativity, the desire to be healthy, and the willingness to be open-minded. Give your body and mind time to adjust and respond.

In addition to retraining your taste buds to enjoy food or drinks without unnatural sugar, oil, and salt, you can do the same when it comes to whole grain bread and pasta. Once you get used to them, you will be surprised to find that you don't miss the white bread and pasta, loaded with an overabundance of starch and sugar and devoid of nutrients. In fact, eventually, you will enjoy the increased richness and more nutty wholesomeness your body learns to yearn for. That's no joke! I see it happen all the time. It happened not only for me but with everyone else I know who switches to a WFPBD. Craving bread, cookies, and other desserts made with whole grains and plant-based options actually replace your old cravings.

Dr. Neal Barnard, a nutritional expert, specializing in diabetes reversal and healthy eating during pregnancy, has saved thousands of patients by introducing them to whole plant-based food. He says, "It only takes about three weeks for our taste buds to change, and then we begin to realize that we don't miss the food we thought we once loved so much." He is absolutely right!

Your Gut Microbiome, Cholesterol, and TMAO

The microbiome, once considered the bacterial environment of our gastrointestinal system (stomach and intestines), was not really understood or discovered until 2006. It consists of thousands and thousands of microorganisms, some "good" and some "bad." Since then, there has been an explosion of research and information coming at the science community, and hopefully, it will be incorporated into our healthcare system soon. It was determined that there are much more than bacteria in our gut; there are also good and bad viruses, yeasts, parasites, and an ancient organism called archaea that has existed for over four billion years in the depths of the oceans and volcanos. It has been found to also reside in our colon. If you follow an unhealthy diet, you will be harboring and feeding more of the bad organisms and vice versa. Everyone's microbiome is different based on what they eat, and yours can be easily converted to a better functioning one with all these organisms living in harmony in a matter of days to weeks on a plant-based eating regimen depending on your current health situation and determination.

In an unhealthy microbiome, the "bad" organisms, along with the liver, create TMAO, the toxic substance produced from the metabolization of carnitine and choline. As we touched on in *Chapter 1*, TMAO production results in the buildup of cholesterol or fat in the inflammatory cells and tissues, causing atherosclerotic plaques in our arteries. People on high-level plant-based diets do not produce TMAO because their microbiomes are balanced with the "good" organisms that dispose of the "bad" organisms and toxins. This is all the more reason to start retraining your taste buds pronto, which you'll soon be doing once you start incorporating the tips outlined in the rest of *Eat Grass, Kick Ass!* Once you do that, your microbiome—and you—will experience the life-changing benefits.

Depending on your personal situation, your healthy diet can begin by cutting out the most dangerous and usual suspects such as fried food, processed food, and drinks containing high fructose corn syrup. If you include sweeteners in your diet, choose whole or minimally processed forms like pureed or whole fruit, date sugar or date syrup, stevia leaves, pure maple syrup, or even pure cane sugar as a starter though cane sugar has very little nutritional value. If you smoke, find a way to stop.

Now, let's start helping you make the switch to a whole food plant-based way of life!

CHAPTER 6

How to Switch To a WFPBD
Hint: Do It Creatively

Prior to switching to a whole food plant-based diet, my husband and our young son insisted that they had some favorite dishes they could not live without. They included white spaghetti noodles, white English muffins, a popular pancake mix, and a syrup made primarily of highly processed fructose corn syrup. Yikes!

We love pancakes, and many times I attempted to teach them about natural syrup being much healthier—pure maple syrup versus the processed stuff. It was an ongoing battle for some years, something they'd enjoy poking fun at me for. Over time, I gradually replaced the eggs, milk, oil, and processed syrup with flax, nondairy milk, and pure maple syrup. I snuck these ingredients into the store-bought containers, starting with a little and working all the way up to 100 percent. While my husband and son made fun of me, I kept my mouth shut until one day when they raved about the pancakes. That made me spill my secret! I broke the news that they had been eating the pure plant products, including maple syrup, for over a year! Ha!

The whole wheat spaghetti pasta and bread transition were more difficult. At first, my family could see and taste the difference when I swapped in the whole grain products for the white ones. For a smoother transition, I started out with just a little whole wheat pasta mixed in with the nonwhole and over the course of the year, I increased to 100 percent. I explained that my goal was to make our meals healthier. When they raved about their spaghetti being so delicious, I informed them that they had been eating 100 percent whole-grain pasta for quite some time. They did a double take, inspecting their food and not believing that it was, in fact, 100 percent whole grain. Granted, their taste buds likely went through a transitional phase, but at least it worked.

The bread was a bit trickier as we had to compromise with lighter wheat bread until the product, Dave's Bread came along. My husband and everyone we know is hooked on that one.

When I converted to my goal of no animal products, my husband saw the changes in me and the benefits to patients I shared whole food plant-based food and information with. Then, as you know from having read the Introduction to this book, he watched *The Game Changers*, and after that, he decided he was ready to go *full-on plant-based*.

So here we are, healthy, happy, functioning at top speed, and feeling great. I love seeing the ever-gleaming sparkle in my husband's eyes as he enjoys his new lease on life thanks to a WFPBD. It's been a great transition for all of us. I was able to make it happen for my family by taking a creative approach. You can make that happen for yourself and your loved ones too.

Eat All You Want on a WFPBD

When switching to a whole food plant-based way of life, take joy in the fact that it will allow you to basically eat as much as you want. Simply put, simple carbohydrates or processed food, lead to weight gain and disease, and complex or unprocessed carbohydrates lead to weight loss and elimination or reduction of cravings, hunger, and disease. Remember, **there are four calories per gram in natural plant food, which contains complex carbohydrates, and nine calories per gram in animal products, which contain no fiber or complex carbohydrates** and a lot of saturated fat, among other dangerous things.

Keep this in mind as you transform your familiar comfort food into healthier, tasty versions as you get on the road to a healthier new you. I will show you how to make the switch with some other amazing tricks I've learned along the way. Begin by eating more of what you know is healthy and less of what you know is unhealthy until you learn to eliminate all, or nearly all, of the bad stuff.

By the way, when people realize you are making significant food choice changes, you will get a variety of reactions. Some will poke fun at you, like my husband and son once did, or try to tell you what they think they know and how you should think. Others will be genuinely curious about your new way of eating, especially because of the new public awareness about the WFPBD. Many will ask you a lot of questions and will be open to your responses. Once you've gotten a pretty good understanding of plant-based eating, I would encourage you to share what you know, help guide others toward appropriate and reliable resources, and be available for any further questions. Lead by example, and then let it go. Focus on your own health and not on trying to change others. Eventually, those around you will see the incredible benefits and come around when they are ready.

Now, let's look at some ways to make the switch to a WFPBD creative and easy.

Tips for Making the Change Easier: Be Kind to Your Body

Avoid, or keep to a minimum, store-bought substitutions for meat and dairy products like cheese, sausage, burgers, etc., until you get good at making your own or learn how to carefully read labels to verify safe and healthy pre-made food selections. Many prepackaged store-bought items are made with fillers, preservatives, and other engineered or processed products. Later, this book will provide you with homemade versions that will be much easier to digest and much healthier for you.

Initially, you may want to incorporate beans by combining them with whole grains (complex carbs) and mild vegetables. As a person's microbiome adjusts, they may experience embarrassing problems like flatulence or burping. Start out with smaller amounts of the beans and increase them gradually. Once your body, or in other words, your microbiome gets used to them, this will improve.

While switching to a WFPBD from a typical American diet, be aware that you may also experience other intestinal issues. New food changes your stomach and intestinal environment, and your gut microbiome will need to rebalance. During the transition, consume a variety of food. For example, don't eat an entire bag of grapes, half of a watermelon, a cup of nuts, a bowl of beans, or a whole box of berries in one sitting. Limit spicy food at first and ease your way back into them. Buffer your stomach with whole-grain bread, cereal, oats, nuts, greens, almonds, sesame seeds, and vegetables, such as potatoes and carrots.

If you're taking blood thinners, use caution with food like green, leafy vegetables and avocados because they can cause imbalances with your blood thinner medications. Your doctor will have to monitor you more closely until you find the right balance in your diet.

You can establish a whole food plant-based lifestyle for your everyday life but may still enjoy some special occasions with holiday food when visiting with family and friends who are not plant-based. A healthy microbiome is not seriously disrupted or changed much with an occasional meal with a small amount of nonplant food. Animals, such as cows, horses, elephants, and apes, with remarkably similar digestive anatomy and processes as humans, occasionally eat tiny amounts of protein in the form of bugs and such. Their microbiome (digestive system) is so well stabilized that it can remove the unwanted protein and fat and flush them out as waste products. It seems only logical that humans can handle a small amount on rare occasions as well. This method has been working well for me! Just do your best to set narrow limits on portions of the unhealthy stuff and try to set a goal of 90 percent or more of plant-based food when filling your plate. Bring your tastiest plant-based dishes to share with people at dinner parties and gatherings. I guarantee that no one will complain.

If you believe you have an addictive-type personality, like many smokers, alcoholics, or fast-food lovers do, you may find it better to be strict and quit your bad food habits entirely once you have established your main food staples. This shouldn't be hard if your everyday kitchen is void of unhealthy food and stocked with plant-based offerings. When you go out to eat, continue to be aware and sensible about your food choices.

Dining Out

Eating at restaurants can be very frustrating. Many times, when I'd order something like a bean burger with whole grain bread or just ask for a salad with hummus and no dairy or meat, the waitstaff would ask, "Do you want to add protein to that?" They don't seem to understand that plants contain protein, especially beans and grains. It drives me crazy when I order a protein bowl without dairy or meat and ask that they add hummus instead of chicken. They frequently remove my avocado and guacamole. "Why did you leave that out?" I ask. They say, "Isn't avocado dairy?" Seriously? This has happened many times. Thankfully, more restaurants are starting to "get it," but it seems to be quite a process everywhere you go. Restaurant owners are beginning to educate their servers on plant-based offerings, and these days you can find quite a few items on the menu to satisfy your plant-based eating lifestyle. You must order correctly and be precise about your preferred ingredients when the staff is modifying a dish to fit your plant-based needs. For example, some fast-food restaurants will make your food dairy-free by replacing cheese and sour cream with pico, salsa, or even veggie cheese. Simply tell the server/waiter/waitress that you are a plant-based eater, meaning you would like the chef to prepare a meal that is dairy-free, meat free, and has dressing on the side or is one made purely of natural products such as balsamic, honey, fruit purées, or mustard. In restaurants, especially finer restaurants, I have found that the wait staff and chef are happy to give personal attention to your plant-based food requests. Most of them enjoy sharing their creative talents and practicing innovative healthy cooking.

As you switch to plant-based eating, teach your children how to find healthy food on a restaurant menu. Before ordering food, gently review the menu choices with them. In the beginning, allow them to choose at will. If you push them, you will likely meet resistance and lose the battle. Encourage them to order a vegetable with every meal and choose broiled or baked food instead of fried.

While allowing children to make selections from the menu, insist that they have at least three colors on their plate. Let them make some mistakes without public embarrassment or confrontation. Afterward, offer reassurance and positive comments at appropriate times. Say how impressed you are that they're taking steps to eat better for a healthier life. Talk to them about the dangers of peer pressure and encourage them to be proud of being a good leader rather than a follower. Gradually phase out nonnutritive food.

And take heart, your new way of eating will save you money when dining out. When you go to a restaurant, the most expensive things on the menu are the filet mignon, steak, lobster, scallops, salmon, and then, usually, the chicken dishes. The veggie stir-fry's, salads, curries, soups, stews, healthy sides, veggie burritos, lasagnas, spaghetti, and such are typically less expensive. A half-gallon of nondairy milk is usually half as costly as cow's milk. The same often goes for butter and eggs. Many plant-based food options are less expensive.

How to Stay on Course at Social Gatherings

At social gatherings where a host or hostess knows that you are a plant-based eater, be sure to tell them that they do not need to make anything special for you. Bring something like a colorful bean salad with a variety of vegetables or a plant-based layered dip. Nuts and seeds are commonly used in plant-based cheese dip replacements, so when you bring food that typically contains nuts or nut butter, consider using seeds instead of nuts. If you use nuts, be considerate by labeling your dish as containing them as many people are severely allergic to them.

For birthday parties, I've found that I can politely request a very thin slice of cake and eat a small bite or none at all. There is no need to take attention away from the celebrant. I just dispose of it later when people are distracted and be sure to fill up beforehand on healthy food so I'm not tempted.

OTHER KEYS TO MAKING THE SWITCH: FASTING, SLEEP, MEDITATION, AND EXERCISE

Fasting

Many nutritional experts recommend a daily fast. When our bodies run out of carbohydrates or glycogen storage, they shift to rely more on our fat storage. Regular fasting for thirteen to fourteen hours allows your body to go into an anaerobic mode to burn old fat stores and cleanse away toxins. For example, a very popular scientifically proven method is to eat dinner early in the evening between four and five o'clock and then eat breakfast at seven or eight the next morning. This is a common practice of Blue Zone populations, those identified as having the healthiest, happiest, longest living populations, whom we encountered earlier in the book, and is very effective for improving and maintaining health.

No one should ever practice fasting for more than a day or two without medical supervision. For those wishing to fast longer than two days to jumpstart a high-level healthy diet, blood pressure can fall dramatically, even for those not on medications. Long term follow-up shows this type of fasting leads to inconsistent benefits. It only works temporarily for those who use it as a bridge to a healthy diet and actually stick to it to make it worth the effort. Extended fasting periods may be useful for cleansing palates and resensitizing or resetting taste buds, making clean food taste good without added salt, butter, oils, soft drinks, and sugar. Again, if you have diabetes or any other underlying condition, consult with your doctor before considering any fasting or changes in diet.

Sleep

Sleep restores damaged cells, especially during REM (rapid eye movement) cycles while repairing the smooth muscles of your internal organs, your heart, and bone tissue, and strengthening your immune system, repairing your eyes, and many other things. Both sleep and exercise play a vital role in reducing stress and improving your level of happiness.

Try to get at least seven and a half hours of sleep at night. Caffeine interferes with sleep and can last long into the late hours. The more you drink, the longer it takes for the half-life to break down to a level that allows your sleep cycles to run as nature intends.

In this fast paced, high stress world which we live, many of us have difficulty with sleeplessness, restlessness, and the resulting anxiety. I myself have long struggled to find ways to increase the amount of sleep I get. "Binaural beats" are a type of scientifically designed music or sounds that can rock your mind to sleep as the tones pass back and forth between the cortexes of your brain. Most are like classical music with steady, consistent, calming sounds. Though many of these studies were done using headsets or earbuds, there are concerns about radiation related to cell phone and earbud use. I find that simply playing the music without these is pretty effective as well. There are many delta binaural beat options available online for sleeping. Look for one with less than 7 hertz. You may have to explore several to find one that works for you. In addition to binaural beats, I find that other calming sounds like white noise, brown noise, pink noise, and even meditation and prayers found on sites that can work as well. Do some research on them and speak with your doctor about his/her suggestions. While listening, it is important to concentrate on taking slow deep breaths to oxygenate the cells of your brain and body. This is also very beneficial for calming your nerves.

Stress and Meditation

Meditation is a very effective way to decrease stress. Stress makes your body release the hormone cortisol, a sugar that can cause massive destruction and damage to nearly every body tissue. In large amounts, it has a significant impact on damaging your heart and your vessels potentially leading to strokes, heart attacks, and many other diseases or disorders. It is essential to recognize this hormonal stress release when it occurs. This is where meditation and exercise come into play. Even better, meditate regularly to help keep stress at controllable levels. Naturally low levels of stress are actually beneficial for motivation and success.

Many scientific studies prove that meditation can significantly improve your health. There are many different meditation styles, from deep breathing and meditation through prayer to practicing yoga techniques, or, in its simplest form, walking in a park or on a beach. Watching a calming movie, reading a book, listening to music, breathing slowly and deeply, and having a relaxing conversation are forms and features of meditation. Practicing yoga or praying helps you focus on a particular activity, thought, object, or goal to clear and calm the mind, bring you peace, and reduce anxiety, depression, and pain.

Exercise

Studies show that physical activity reverses brain shrinkage, improves memory, and decreases mortality by 50 percent. Nutritional experts commonly recommend that you get at least three and a half hours of exercise per week or twenty to thirty minutes of walking per day. Just breaking a sweat on a regular basis can remove toxins from your body and improve skin and complexion. Endorphins are happy hormones that are released with exercise and can relieve stress, elevate your mood, and reduce frustration. Weight-bearing exercise is of equal importance for keeping your bones and joints healthy and strong. To build up strength, try doing push-ups on an incline with your hands on a chair or on the stairs and do squats or lunges for leg strengthening. Many people with heart conditions who have a limited ability to walk even a few feet can reverse their heart disease and increase their ability to walk or even run for miles after just a couple of weeks on strict whole food plant-based diets. See Dr. Dean Ornish's Nutrition as Medicine Lifestyle Programs now supported by our government through Medicare. Also, check out the free 21-Day jumpstart program offered by Dr. Neal Barnard on his site at https://kickstart.pcrm.org.

Choose the Right Drinks

Daily drink choices are important, and since your body is made up of about 60 percent water, that should be your primary drink. If you enjoy soft drinks or soda, the American Heart Association recommendation is less than one soft drink per day. That's not very many. Plenty of studies show the unhealthy effects of soft drinks, mostly because of the amount and type of sugar. Many have high fructose corn syrup, and the zero-calorie sugar replacements are often just as bad. Soft drinks usually include chemicals for coloring, artificial flavors, and chemicals designed to keep you hooked on them.

Even healthier sweeteners like maple syrup, honey, and pure cane sugar are cumulatively addictive, so it is best to retrain your taste buds to enjoy lower sugar, and better yet, unsweetened beverages. Many artificial colors and preservatives are known to aggravate conditions such as asthma, skin hives, rashes, blemishes, allergies, and depression, all of which have been associated with high soft drink intake. A great way to replace soft drinks is to add lemon, cucumber, pure fruit juice, or mint to water. Mint is very easy to grow indoors, by the way. You can also add a small amount of 100 percent pure blended fruit juice to flavor your water.

Less than three cups per day of organic, decaf or moderately caffeinated coffee has shown many health benefits. Coffee beans contain protective plant polyphenol compounds that lower your blood pressure. The caffeine in coffee can elevate energy levels, resulting in more exercise and movement, has some protective effects on the liver in chronic hepatitis patients and it can sharpen the mind. As previously mentioned, caffeine can have detrimental effects on our sleep patterns and also on developing babies and children. Organic tea from natural herbs and spices can also provide many health benefits.

If you drink a lot of coffee, it will take some time to wean down to a more healthy and manageable level. Try cutting your coffee in half with more water or drink decaf coffee, which still contains about 25 percent caffeine, or try adding some nondairy milk or nondairy creamer to replace some coffee. You can make homemade oat milk creamer by simply blending rolled oats with water, making it delicious and *heart-healthy*. You may even find it available in your local store.

Parting Words

As you switch to a WFPBD, I'm confident you'll start to love your new lifestyle and the new you that will result. Keep your goal in mind—whether it be reversing or managing disease, improving overall health, seeking a slimmer body, or all of the above, stick with your plan. Every second of the effort and energy you put into this will be well worth it!

CHAPTER 7

Tips and Tricks: Making Whole Plant-Based Food Preparation Easier and Healthier

It is said that peer pressure is the number one reason people don't stick to a healthy diet. My years as a nurse has led me to the conclusion that the reason people do not stick to a healthy diet goes deeper than merely peer pressure. I observed that people often continue to eat in an unhealthy manner because they don't know how to replace the food that is ingrained in their family culture and traditions. They don't have reliable nutrition information or the awareness of the many natural alternatives for creating healthy dishes that would comply with their culture and traditions.

So let's examine how to make whole food plant-based dish preparation easier and healthier.

Add Green, Leafy Vegetables and Legumes to Everything Possible

Start by adding green, leafy vegetables and legumes (beans, peas, and lentils) to as many things as possible, like spaghetti sauce, soups, stews, pasta dishes, and grain dishes. Green, leafy vegetables contain calcium, iron, folate, and fiber and are low in calories. They decrease inflammation, help food move through your intestines, improve eyesight, balance cholesterol levels, enhance skin, fight cancer, promote weight loss, boost energy, and increase lifespan.

Incorporate leafy greens into smoothies - don't be afraid to blend in some spinach or kale. Often no one even knows it is in there. A handful of spinach virtually disappears and is tasteless in smoothies that are colored with berries or cocoa and is packed with nutrients. If possible, try to maintain a 60/40 ratio of vegetables and fruit throughout your day—more vegetables than fruit.

Cook or steam your vegetables with low sodium vegetable stock, broth, or water. It is not necessary to fry or cook them or anything in oil, especially for those with cholesterol concerns. Steaming vegetables helps to ensure you to retain all the nutrients and is preferable to boiling, straining, and losing these nutrients.

Greens preservation Tip: To make your greens last longer and save space in your refrigerator, snip the ends of your cilantro, parsley, lettuce heads, etc., and place them in water in a shallow gravy boat or bowl on the counter near your sink and change the water daily. Surprisingly, they can last longer and look more beautiful that way.

Add Herbs and Spices

Many plant-based eaters love hot, spicy sauces to "make everything taste good." They put them and other favorite herbs and spices on plant-based eggs and cheese, pasta, noodles, and any new, unfamiliar food until they come around to appreciating the change to healthier food.

For those hot pepper lovers out there, freeze those babies whole. When ready to use, pull one out of the freezer and slice it right away rather than defrost it, which will make it mushy. When they're frozen, you'll have less capsaicin pepper juice on your hands and cutting boards and less risk of those burning oils soaking into your fingers and getting into your eyes. They slice up beautifully to top favorites like avocado toast, veggie pizza, finger food, and other appetizers.

(Time Saver) Prepare Meals Ahead

Make extra lasagna, spaghetti sauce, soups, and stews to freeze in portion sizes to have on hand for quick lunches or for meals on days when cooking is just not an enjoyable or possible feat.

Make your homemade plant-based versions of burgers, mayonnaise, cheese, sauces, sour cream, dressings, etc., weekly or on a four-month basis to be refrigerated or frozen and have on hand when needed. Freeze whole grain buns, bread, or dough, and thaw a loaf as needed.

You can prepare meal ingredients ahead of time, place them in the refrigerator or freezer, and then transfer them to a crockpot to turn on in the morning to be ready when you arrive home.

Involve your family in preparing meals as this will increase their enjoyment of trying new things and encourage them to give input. Spending time with family is so important. As the old saying goes, "The family that plays together stays together." Or, in this case, "The family that cooks together stays together."

(Money Saver) Buy Grains, Beans, Flour, and Rice in Bulk

People believe eating plant-based food is expensive, but it really isn't. Many of the plants highest in protein come in the form of beans or grains (canned, dried, or frozen) and are available in bulk. Consider using dry beans and purchase them in large quantities. You will save a lot of money and get a nutrition-packed bean without the added salt and the toxins from the cans. Store your grains, flours, and rice in airtight containers in cool dark cabinets to preserve quality and freshness.

Bean Preparation

When preparing dry beans, soak, cook, and rinse them as recommended to reduce their lectin content. Lectin is a carbohydrate-binding protein found in almost all food but especially in legumes and grains. High amounts of it can cause severe gastrointestinal illnesses. Low levels of lectins are actually a healthy addition to your diet and act as antioxidants protecting cells from damage. Wheat germ lectin found in whole wheat has been shown to fight cancer, especially tumors related to colorectal cancer. They also slow digestion and slow the absorption of carbohydrates, preventing spikes in blood sugar levels thereby reducing diabetes complications. Foods containing lectins are also associated with lower cardiovascular disease and lower body weight.

Consider preparing your own beans from dried ones bought in bulk rather than using canned beans to avoid additives like salt or the potential leaching of industrial chemicals like those from container liners with bisphenol A (BPA). When buying cans or bottles of food, people tend to look for the "non-BPA lining" label. Dr. Michael Greger's research exposes that many products that have had the BPA toxin removed have, in its place, other chemicals like bisphenol S (BPS) and bisphenol F (BPF), which are very similar to BPA and have a similar effect on the body, including hormone disruption, problems with reproduction, metabolism, and neurological function. Food regulation boards state that BPA levels remaining in product containers are safe for human consumption. Research shows that these chemicals are potentially harmful but are unavoidable as they are found in and on many other sources such as water bottles and store receipts.

To be on the safer side, choose fresh, frozen, or dried food over canned food whenever possible. When using plastic containers for food and drinks, don't put them in the microwave or dishwasher, and don't leave them in plastic containers in a hot car. Glass, ceramic, and stainless-steel containers are considered the safest to use.

(Time Saver) Clean and Rinse as You Go

One great thing about plant-based food is that you don't have to worry about contamination from dangerous germs or diseases that meat can leave behind on your cutting boards or countertops. Cleaning up is extremely easy. Be sure to wash all of your store-bought produce well, even if they are labeled as "pre-rinsed" or "prewashed." Rice and grains, including quinoa, must be rinsed well and cooked properly to remove saponins, an animal deterrent chemical that causes digestive problems, and other potential toxins/antinutrients. Rinse your cooking supplies right away after using them to save you from extra work. When working with washed vegetables and the dishes look clean, you really only need to rinse them. Of course, you must continue to wash any items people eat from, such as utensils and dishes.

(Waste Reduction) Freeze or Can Everything You Don't Use within a Week

We never let bananas turn brown in our home and go to waste. We peel and freeze them to make delicious smoothies, snacks, bread, and ice cream. You can also substitute bananas for eggs, oil, butter, and sugar wherever a sweet banana flavor is acceptable. Bananas are high in fiber, potassium, calcium, and prebiotics, which are gut-friendly food for the good microorganisms that induce growth or activity of live beneficial bacterial organisms, known as probiotics. Bananas help reduce acid reflux, lower high blood pressure, reduce depression, prevent bloating, and aid in bowel movement regulation.

Store-bought "fresh" fruit and vegetables are picked before they can ripen on the vine and often weeks before they arrive in stores, which can prevent them from reaching their nutritional potential. Frozen fruit and vegetables are allowed to ripen naturally and are picked at the peak of ripeness, then flash-frozen, which locks in the nutrients. You can buy them in bulk at great prices, and they usually have the most flavor.

Before any fruit or vegetables go bad, wash, dry, slice, and place them in baggies or containers, then put them in the freezer and use them within the next few weeks. It is very easy to freeze all kinds of vegetables, including bell peppers, eggplant, zucchini, mushrooms, spinach, Swiss chard, kale, and chunks of beets or ginger.

Ginger is a delicious addition to stir-fry dishes. Freezing portion cut pieces of unpeeled ginger wrapped in plastic wrap or baggies will change your life. When ready to use, allow it to thaw for a few minutes on the counter, rub off or cut off the outer peel, then slice it or mince it. You will not run out of ginger again, nor will you have those large roots shriveling up in your fruit bowls before you can use them. You can do the same with peeled garlic to have on hand.

If growing basil, parsley, or mint, don't let it go to waste either as summer comes to a close. Turn it into pesto to freeze for future pasta, grain bowls, and bread spreads, and have it on hand for adding fresh, healthy flavor to anything else you can think of.

A variety of colorful whole fruit and berries are rich in antioxidants, fiber, and nutrients and have low glycemic indexes, making them an excellent sweetener and source for fighting cancer, heart disease, and diabetes. Add them to your oatmeal, cereal, and smoothies for a great way to start your day. Frozen banana and berries are delicious in smoothies. Add fruit and berries to water to enhance flavor, increase your intake, and flush toxins from your body. Add fruit and berries when baking muffins, cookies, and cakes. Cook them to create delicious compotes, purees, jams, and sauces for use on toast, in ice cream, or in other desserts.

Line Your Pans with Parchment Paper

Parchment paper is a nonstick, heat- and burn-resistant baking paper that is quite handy when baking tofu, cookies, or roasting vegetables. It definitely cuts down on cleaning. Baking mats made from food-safe silicone can also be used quickly and easily with minimal cleanup.

Use Nonstick, Versatile Cookware

Boncook, formerly known as DeMarle at Home, is a fantastic cookware product that I have stocked up on over the years. It is very popular in high-end restaurants, especially in Europe, for making consistently beautiful loaves of bread, desserts, pastries, muffins, cakes, crustless quiches, etc. Rarely does anything stick to these products, so you can easily and quickly rinse them, wash them with warm, soapy water, or place them in the dishwasher. They are safe in the oven up to 475 degrees. They are made from food-safe silicone, containing crushed, spun glass that makes food crispy on the outside. This flexible bakeware comes in every shape and size you could ever think of and has amazing nonstick properties. Shapes include fancy designed one-piece Bundt pan, loaf pans (many sizes), muffin cups (many sizes), rolls, cake pans, pie pans, etc. This is not a sales pitch for the company. I am just sharing what I feel is an incredible product that has made my life so much more fun and easier. It is very difficult to find anything comparable, even in kitchen specialty stores.

Meal Replacements On the Run

It is best to eat whole plant food, but sometimes it just doesn't seem possible. This is especially true for young adults in college and those working long, high-stressed, fast-paced, fourteen-hour or longer shifts, like doctors, nurses, and resident medical students.

My two daughters, Lauren and Heather, have always been very aware of healthy food and the importance of exercise, but while they were in college, demanding schedules and peer pressure often made healthy eating difficult. They were in a continual study mode, and roommates and others would often bring around junk food, especially at their most vulnerable moments. When I got wind of this, I realized I needed to step in and help my daughters, so I began sending them a bit of health insurance magic in the mail. Read on.

For situations like college students encounter, it is good to have a quick meal on hand to make in a matter of seconds without needing a blender. I am not referring to the popular protein shakes because isolated protein powders or, again, isolated anything that removes parts of a plant's natural composition results in health consequences. I'm talking about powdered meals. Check the label to confirm it contains whole plant ingredients. Even though a powdered meal contains ingredients not in their natural form, some meal replacement powders are "plant-based" and can include everything the original whole food contains, including the fiber, nutrients, and protein. The only thing that seems to be missing is the water. It is so easy to grab a shaker cup and some meal replacement powder before running out the door.

Meal replacement powder may seem a bit pricey at first, but when you calculate the number of meals you get from a container, they usually cost less than three dollars per meal. You can't beat that price even at a fast-food restaurant. I justify an occasional dried meal replacement powder because of the time it saves in the kitchen and because it benefits your health over the fast-food alternatives, which really aren't that fast anyway with the commute, frustrations of finding healthy food, and ordering and communication problems involved. Just make sure you read the labels carefully and select the healthiest product you can find.

I learned about the importance of having these healthy backup meals from my friends, who always seemed amazingly healthy and fit, even soon after having babies. I would eat my healthy food and exercise like crazy six times a week and still carried an extra fifteen pounds. At parties and other gatherings, these gals always amazed me with their self-control when desserts were around. After some probing, they admitted to having plant-based meal shakes beforehand! But pleasantly surprising to me, my weight has stayed down without it since going full-on plant-based.

Grow Your Own Food, Indoors and Out

Indoor gardening can be a wonderful experience for people of all ages. There is nothing quite like having fresh homegrown herbs and vegetables at your fingertips. You can easily find what you need at garden centers and online for growing most of your cooking essentials indoors. These include garlic, ginger, green onions, cilantro, parsley, mint, romaine, spinach, and shallots, just to name a few. Having an indoor garden is a fantastic learning experience for children and one of the things I cherish most that my parents passed on to my siblings and me. I'll tell that story in some detail later in the book.

Some quick tips are to set up your indoor garden in a south-facing window, if you can, or use grow lights. Be sure to use a good potting mix with vermiculite for adequate drainage. Most plants need plant food on a monthly basis and water regularly when dry to the touch or just before wilting, depending on the plant and the recommendations.

For the most benefit to your health and the environment, use nontoxic, natural insecticides like diatomaceous earth, neem oil, mint oils, and rosemary oils mixed with water and a little soap rather than those toxic pesticides that make you wait so many days before you can "safely" pick and eat your food.

Outdoor gardening is another fantastic experience for adults and children. There is nothing like being outside in the fresh air, working the earth in the sunshine, and obtaining the super healthy benefits of vitamin D. The sun provides a better form of vitamin D than supplements do, though your location and the time of year can considerably impact the levels you acquire. It is easy enough to have your doctor check your vitamin D levels to determine your needs. If the sun is plentiful in your area, all you will require is about ten to fifteen minutes per day over your arms and face while gardening or walking outdoors. If you are at risk for skin cancer, be sure to protect yourself.

If you have a small yard and want to have your garden up and away from critters and pests or just want to prevent a bad back, create a raised garden or boxed garden. It is nice to have your herbs at an easy-to-grab height and easy-to-weed level. You can build a raised garden yourself by using wood, filter cloth, and quarter-inch square fence wire on the bottom to keep grubs and ground critters from getting into your garden. Use good soil, including mushroom compost, and ensure proper drainage and nutrients. There are plenty of resources online for creating your own boxed or raised gardens.

If you have some space, and depending on your climate zone, consider planting a fruit tree or two. Choose a popular favorite like the Belle of Georgia peach tree with peaches so sweet and delicious the juice drips down your chin as you bite into it. Thinking about this takes me back to my childhood. Two other popular and delicious fruit trees to grow are Honeycrisp and Gala apple trees or plum trees like South Dakota, Santa Rosa, Stanley, or Seneca. Consider planting a Medjool date tree as well, which will be quite handy for many plant-based recipes. Most trees do well in climate zones 4-8. Check to make sure your climate will sustain whichever species you select.

Keep Moving Forward

As you implement the tricks and tips in this chapter to make your food preparation easier and healthier, remember that the effort is worth it for your health and overall outlook. Anything worth having requires discipline and work to achieve. Keep that in mind as you keep moving forward!

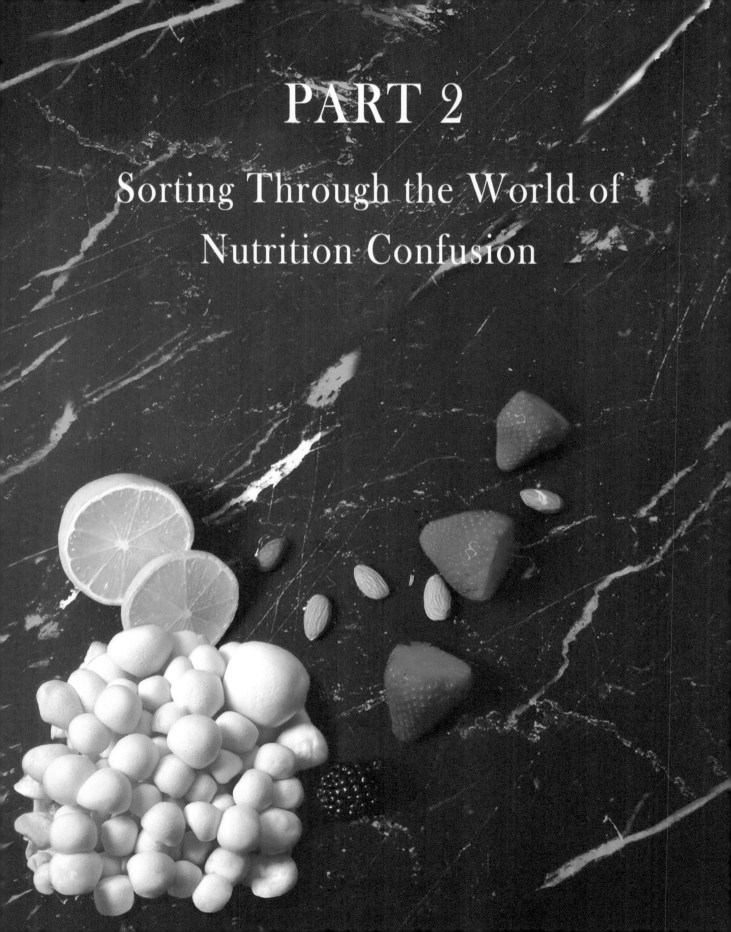

PART 2

Sorting Through the World of Nutrition Confusion

CHAPTER 8

Science and Research: How to Seek and Find the Truth

A general Internet search for health information will not produce the most accurate results. The amount of misinformation on the Internet is mindboggling, with the vast majority of the news articles on nutrition containing inaccurate information. Awareness and frustration with this fact are a common theme at nutritional medicine healthcare conferences I've attended over the years. Yet, many of these online sources are ones that people tend to feel they can trust.

For example, when searching for the "best source of protein", meat and dairy products are usually suggested first. What these information providers fail to tell you, or what they don't know is that these sources are too high in the amount of protein and they are the wrong type of protein for our bodies. These proteins including carnitine, casein, choline, and IGF-1, have been proven to cause the most common inflammatory diseases in America. Adding to the confusion in research studies and Internet searches over the years is the language and the definition of terms used to describe different types of diets and other related data evolve or change, making it more difficult for the public to interpret older scientific study data and compare it to newer studies.

That said, the most confusing and possibly dangerous source of information the public receives is through media outlets that tend to provide misinformation in the form of fact cover-ups, cherry-picked, hyped-up, false headlines, and stories full of inaccurate details for a partisan gain. For instance, some news sources quickly attack films such as "The Game Changers," the documentary which describes the benefits of a plant-based diet. These news sources pull details out of context to hyperinflate their stories to find ways to defend the continued eating of animal products without regard for the damage they are causing the public. Their sole focus is monetary gain and they are often controlled by the industries that own or support them.

Sadly, many well-intentioned nutritionists, doctors, nurses, and other trusted specialists often blindly promote the media's misinformation, ingraining it as "truth" in the public's mind. Fortunately, the public has access to a great deal of scientific data on websites such as that of the National Institutes of Health which is responsible for biomedical and public health research, but this data often requires extensive training and knowledge in order for data to be properly interpreted.

Examining the Studies

Another factor, and perhaps one of the most important in determining the legitimacy and accuracy of studies, is to have a clear understanding of potential conflicts of interest. This is critical in determining if results are interpreted free of funding bias, a key signal that the study results should be highly questioned. Knowing who conducted the studies, what industries or related individuals may benefit, determining if there is an agenda or special interest, when the studies were done compared to other or previous study data, making sure no information is ignored or left out intentionally, and whether language may be used to sway readers' perceptions are all things to consider.

An example of funding bias is shown in a study by the *Journal of the American College of Cardiology*. Without even looking at the title, seeing that it is from a heart journal, the average medical and nonmedical person may already assume the study is legitimate because of where it appears, right?

The title is "Saturated Fats and Health: A Reassessment and Proposal for Food-based Recommendations: JACC State-of-the-Art Review." The footnotes section states that the funding was from a "non-partisan, educational organization

whose primary goal is to ensure US nutrition policy based on rigorous scientific evidence." Following that statement are the names and disclosures of about eleven contributors, three of whom have nothing to disclose. The other eight contributors, however, declare a long list showing that they are speakers for and on boards for milk foundations, national beef associations, pharmaceutical companies, milk producer educational programs, dairy farmers' committees and management, and Nestlé and General Mills—both very powerful processed food distributors.

If I were one of the three individuals or entities without anything to disclose, perhaps one who had no affiliation with any mighty meat or dairy industry, I would feel significantly outweighed in representation in that room. In the journal abstract, they state: "Whole-fat dairy, unprocessed meat, eggs, and dark chocolate are SFA (saturated fatty acid)-rich food with a complex matrix that is not associated with increased risk of CVD (cardiovascular disease). The totality of available evidence does not support further limiting the intake of such food." This goes completely against what most of us have known or have been told for many years. We have seen with our own eyes that people who have eliminated saturated fat from their diets show the contrary in lab results. Even more maddening is watching journalists run with studies such as this, creating headlines, hype stories, more frustration, confusion, and disinformation in the public's minds. This type of reporting leads many people to distrust anything they hear about nutrition and simply give up.

Perhaps the biggest problem of all is that the scientists who perform the research and know the truth are not the ones with big money paying to disseminate the information to the public. The industries, their lawyers, privately paid (either direct or indirect) scientists, and doctors are hired to wrongly "verify" biased, agenda-driven misinformation. We have been inundated with this througout our lives and are brainwashed to a great extent. Clear evidence of this is in the commercials we are exposed to on television. There are basically two large industries drilling our brain every time we watch it. One is the food industry showing commercial after commercial of juice dripping from cheesy grilled burgers and oil laden fried food; the other is the pharmaceutical industry pushing tons of medications to treat all the inflammatory diseases caused by those foods in the commercials. Fortunately, there are scientists who have been continuously working most of their careers to stop the lies and these dangerous ads through court. They have also been treating their happy patients with great success and doing their best to educate the public.

Closing Thoughts

Quality information about health and nutrition can only be found if you know where to look. Most legitimate studies are done using strict scientific research methods, and reports will include all of the data used to determine the findings, not just pieces of it. The average person and many medical professionals don't have the time, training, or experience to decipher this complex data. There are many studies the general public does not have access to. Some studies are available in their entirety and there are many in brief abstracts online, but often you have to have approval for direct access to download entire studies or must pay a fee to see the data and results.

For an awe-inspiring glimpse of one who has spent his life studying and clarifying study research data, watch Dr. Michael Greger at NutritionFacts.org. His video *Food as Medicine: Preventing & Treating the Most Common Diseases with Diet* can be easily found online.

Plenty of doctors on TV and social media are thought to be experts on health and nutrition, but none are as specialized in the science behind health and nutrition and make themselves as freely accessible as Dr. Greger. He thoroughly evaluates nutritional health studies in the archives of the US National Library of Medicine at the National Institutes of Health, known as PubMed or Medline, and other study databases around the world. He has scrutinized hundreds of thousands of research studies, combing through them for accuracy, turning gray areas into black and white. He is extremely well-respected, regarded as a leading expert in deciphering the purest of answers for health-and nutrition-related questions, and he does it as a free service for all humankind[33].

At conferences around the world, he is famously known for his opening quote, "Every year I read through every issue of every English-language nutrition journal in the world so busy folks like you don't have to." He encourages people to share his findings to help in his quest to improve health through accurate information worldwide.

I have had the honor and pleasure of attending many conferences with numerous plant-based nutrition experts who are all in the same spectrum of truth in nutrition and health as Dr. Greger, meaning they are all whole food plant-based supporters. They are incredibly impressive speakers all around the world and can be found on the internet. Their hearts are set on sharing the truth and spreading this information through education and changing public policy to benefit all. They ask for nothing in return except continued support in spreading the word. You will meet more of these legendary nutritional experts in the next chapter.

CHAPTER 9

Excellent Resources:
The World's Leading Whole Food Plant-Based Doctors

Who to Trust ... Pulling It All Together

As a nurse, I have struggled with a perplexing question over the years: Why do most doctors use medication as the first line of treatment when it is clear that they are merely treating the symptoms and not the cause? Many doctors report that most patients would rather take medicine because they don't understand how to make a positive dietary switch from their lifelong eating habits. Some doctors admit that they are afraid to prescribe a new eating plan for fear that something will go wrong if their patients cannot commit to it. Many other doctors say that they simply don't have the proper nutrition education background to guide their patients in a natural way to adequately address poor health conditions.

Additionally, few doctors have the time, level, or type of expertise required to decipher accurate nutrition information from the enormous libraries of complex research studies. I hold the utmost respect for these hard-working healthcare professionals who find that they are limited and driven by a system that often feels entirely out of control. With the ever-growing population and the limited number of doctors, the problem is getting worse. But for the general public looking for the right answers, narrowing in on the specialists who have dedicated their lives and expertise in the field of nutrition is an enormous benefit.

Then comes the most frequent question I am asked today: Who can I believe and who can you trust? With all the conflicting information out there, people really don't know who to trust. For many years, I asked the same question.

There are some medical research experts however, who critically examine studies, compare results, and provide an analytical review and summary of them. They are high-level critical thinkers that have a firm understanding and can interpret health science for us in a nonbiased, truthful, and understandable way. That is where Dr. Michael Greger and other nutritional experts, many of whom you've already encountered in this book, come in. In this chapter, you will learn more about them. They have dedicated their lives to putting out health data in lay terms, and for decades have fought battles trying to get the truth out in the midst of massive misinformation propagated by the powerful pharmaceutical, meat, and dairy organizations. The expertise of these scientists in dealing with them is precisely what we need.

Discovering the Truth: The Scientists Who Really Know

In 2011, I found the fountain of truth. That year, I discovered these scientists who, for many decades, had devoted their lives to uncovering the connection between nutrition and health. My first Nutrition as Medicine conference confirmed that the people on stage were the top nutritional health doctors and scientists in the world, all who mutually supported the free sharing of nutritional health information "simply as a service to humanity". The fact that they clearly had no agenda led me to many more of their conferences and other plant-based study programs.

More on Dr. Michael Greger

Of all the extremely impressive experts behind the science of nutrition, I mention Dr. Greger most frequently because he is a nutritional research ROCKSTAR! His site, NutritionFacts.org, is a fountain of knowledge where he has created free informational programs loaded with excellent video clips on nearly every health and nutrition subject you can think of. At speaking engagements, the standing ovations and cheers from his audience are extraordinary and his popularity extends to Europe and Australia, in addition to the US.

His website is easy to navigate and functions as a noncommercial, nonprofit, science-based public service provided by Dr. Greger himself. He gives "daily updates on the latest in nutrition research via bite-sized videos" and answers questions with accurate, trustworthy, and up-to-date information. You simply input any search criteria to receive a thorough, fact-based review of studies on any nutrition-related subject.

Nutritional data and information is expanding greatly so be aware that particularly since 2006, a flood of information has been reported through many studies with the discovery of TMAO and its effect on our microbiome. There is often a lag time of about 17 years for scientific studies to be processed, completed, and disseminated in a manner that has an effect within the medical community, and transmitted to the public. He encourages people to let him know if his site lacks any topic. He is committed to addressing such issues right away. He asks that people first check PubMed.ncbi.nlm.nih.gov (Medline) and look for some research on the subject before bringing it to his attention. He will thoroughly evaluate the studies and try to include his evaluation on his next daily podcast.

Dr. Greger's interest in the nutrition field has earnest beginnings. As a child in the '70s, he saw how his grandmother, who had been sent home to die, was saved by Dr. Nathan Pritikin and his plant-based food program. At the age of sixty-five, she was confined to a wheelchair with end-stage heart disease and crushing chest pain. By changing her diet, she reversed her heart disease and became fully functional, walking ten miles a day in only three weeks. She became a star patient of Dr. Pritikin's.

Mrs. Greger lived for thirty-one more years to the age of ninety-six on a plant-based diet and lifestyle program. As a result of Dr. Greger's grandmother's experience, he became a doctor and an expert in interpreting nutritional data studies over the past sixty years or so. To honor his grandmother, and as a free service to humanity, he makes himself available to answer all questions related to health and nutrition and creates a clear picture for the general public around the globe.

One of my favorite quotes from Dr. Greger, first heard at a healthcare conference, goes, "Sure, you could choose moderation and hit yourself with a smaller hammer. But why beat yourself up at all?" Isn't that the truth! To get and stay healthy, you have to embrace a healthy lifestyle.

Dr. Greger was invited as an expert witness in defense of Oprah Winfrey at the infamous "meat defamation" trial. He lectures at the Conference on World Affairs and the National Institutes of Health and has appeared as a special guest on shows such as *The Colbert Report* and *The Dr. Oz Show*. Dr. Greger authored the books *How Not to Diet* and *The How Not to Die Cookbook* based on whole plant-based food and detailed scientific study data, which became an instant *New York Times* Bestseller. He also authored *Carbophobia: The Scary Truth Behind America's Low Carb Craze*, where he draws together decades of research with hundreds of reputable resources exposing the dangerous truth behind low-carb diets.

He offers clarity over confusion and supports the foundational principles of healthy eating and healthy living. Dr. Greger donates to charity all speaking fees and proceeds he receives from his books and DVDs.

Dr. Greger developed what he calls the Daily Dozen recommendations—I'll go into some detail about this in a minute—for which he has teams of volunteers who have helped him create and maintain an app for tracking.

He is very easy to find online doing free interviews for public benefit, and he publishes a daily video podcast to address people's questions that you can subscribe to for free at Nutritionfacts.org. He performs all of this work through his nonprofit organization and is not influenced by industry, lobbyists, or other commercial organizations. As for the Daily Dozen, it is a checklist of all the things he recommends you try to fit into a daily routine. He classifies food and activities as shown in abbreviated form in the list that follows. I've omitted the serving sizes and a lot of valuable information supporting this because I feel they are somewhat complicated for the purpose of this book, but you can easily find the details if you go to Dr. Greger's online sources or his books *How Not to Diet*, *How Not to Die*, and *Discover the Foods Scientifically Proven to Prevent and Reverse Disease*. The main idea is to get a variety of food from each of these categories each day. You will find that this is easy to do on a whole food plant-based diet.

1. *Legumes (beans, peas, and lentils)* – Black beans, black-eyed peas, butter beans, cannellini beans, split peas, chickpeas, lentils, pea soup, hummus, edamame, English peas, great northern beans, kidney beans, small red beans, and tempeh.

2. *Berries* – Blackberries, blueberries, raspberries (black and red), strawberries, cherries, acai berries, barberries, concord grapes, raisins, cranberries, goji berries, kumquats, and mulberries.

3. *Other Fruit* – Apples, dried apricots, avocados, bananas, dates, mangos, cantaloupes, clementine's, nectarines, oranges, grapefruits, kiwis, lemons, limes, watermelons, peaches, pears, pineapples, papayas, passion fruits, dried figs, honeydews, plums, pomegranates, prunes, lychees, and pluots.

4. *Cruciferous Vegetables* – Arugula, Brussels sprouts, bok choy, broccoli, cabbage, cauliflower, collards, horseradish, kale, mustard greens, radishes, turnip greens, and watercress.

5. *Greens* – Arugula, beet greens, collard greens, kale, mesclun mix, mustard greens, sorrel, spinach, Swiss chard, and turnip greens.

6. *Other Vegetables* – Artichokes, asparagus, beets, bell peppers, carrots, corn, garlic, green beans, string beans, mushrooms (button, oyster, portobello, and shiitake), okra, onions, purple potatoes, pumpkin, sea vegetables (dulse, arame, and nori), snap peas, squash (delicata, summer, and spaghetti), sweet potatoes/yams, tomatoes, and zucchini.

7. *Flaxseeds* – Golden or brown, crushed.

8. *Nuts and Seeds* – Almonds, Brazil nuts, cashews, chia seeds, hazelnuts/filbert, hemp seeds, macadamia nuts, peanuts, pecans, pistachios, pumpkin seeds, sesame seeds, sunflower seeds, and walnuts.

9. *Herbs and Spices*– Allspice, barberries, basil, bay leaves, cardamom, chili powder, cilantro, cinnamon, cloves, coriander, cumin, curry powder, dill, fenugreek, garlic, ginger, horseradish, lemongrass, marjoram, mustard powder, nutmeg, oregano, smoked paprika, parsley, pepper, peppermint, rosemary, saffron, sage, thyme, turmeric, and vanilla.

10. *Whole Grains* – Barley, brown rice, buckwheat, millet, oats, popcorn, quinoa, rye, teff, whole-wheat flour, whole wheat pasta, and wild rice.

11. *Organic Beverages* – Black tea, chai tea, vanilla, chamomile tea, coffee, Earl Grey tea, green tea, hibiscus tea, hot chocolate, jasmine tea, lemon balm tea, matcha tea, almond blossom oolong tea, peppermint tea, rooibos tea, water, and white tea.

12. *Exercise* - All exercise, including moderate activities like yard work, walking briskly, biking, swimming, hiking, doubles tennis, and more vigorous activities like jogging, rock climbing, circuit weight training, running, singles tennis, football.

Dr. T. Colin Campbell

As mentioned in Chapter 2, Dr. Campbell is recognized as one of the earliest pioneers of the plant-based movement. He is credited for labeling the term "plant-based diet" in 1980. He wanted to distinguish the impact of low-fat, high-fiber, whole-vegetable-based food on cancer and to separate this type of diet from the terms "vegetarian" and "vegan." Dr. Campbell does not identify as a vegetarian or a vegan because he says, "they often infer something other than what I espouse."

In 1965, armed with a doctorate degree in nutrition, biochemistry, and microbiology, Dr. T. Colin Campbell worked for the State Department in the Philippines developing a network of feeding centers to ensure that malnourished children consumed adequate protein. He was a huge part of the discovery of a strong link between animal protein and cancer. Dr. Campbell's findings were so compelling that he received grants for roughly seventy years of research from Oxford and Cornell, the National Cancer Institute, the Chinese government, and the UK Imperial Cancer Research Fund. He found remarkably consistent evidence regarding the dangers of animal protein consumption.

He has authored more than 300 research papers and several books, including *The China Study: Startling Implications for Diet* and *Weight Loss and Long-term Health*, which has sold more than two million copies worldwide. It is one of the most comprehensive studies of health and nutrition ever conducted. He has been featured in many documentary films such as *Forks over Knives*, *Eating You Alive*, *Food Matters*, and *PlantPure Nation*. He has been on expert panels for the United States National Academy of Sciences on food safety since 1978. He continues to share his time traveling as a guest speaker at many conferences, even well into his eighties and is a regular contributor of articles for Naked Food Magazine sharing his expertise on a whole food plant-based diet around the world.

The China Study was a twenty-year effort that examined the link between the consumption of animal products and chronic illnesses, such as heart disease, diabetes, and various types of cancer. Dr. Campbell found a dramatic connection between casein, the main protein in dairy milk and liver cancer. *The New York Times* described it as "the Grand Prix of Epidemiology." The study concluded that the geographical areas where people consumed more animal-based food were more likely to have higher death rates from Western-diet type diseases, while the opposite was true of plant-based food.

Many doctors will tell you that they received very little to no nutrition education through medical school and say that they are horrified when they finally get around to reading *The China Study.* They report a "feeling of a lot of guilt" for having practiced medicine poorly all those years. For genuine, heartfelt reactions to what these doctors learn, see *PlantPure Nation*, the movie at Plantpurenation.com. It is an absolute eye-opener and will help you understand why there is so much controversy over food and diets.

Dr. Campbell states that one of the biggest concerns today is that more than 50 percent of Americans now have type 2 diabetes, and at least 93 percent of these cases are preventable. He confirms that we should not be relying on the idea that genes are the determinants of our health and that it is a matter of turning off the genes with what we eat and changing lifestyle habits. This is clearly demonstrated with gene mapping images he shares during his lectures at conferences showing how this works.

He also declares that "the 'War on Cancer' is failing as professionals continue to ignore the connection to animal protein" and that "there are virtually no nutrients in animal-based food that are not better provided by plants."

Learn more about Dr. Campbell at Nutritionstudies.org.

Dr. Caldwell Esselstyn

Dr. Caldwell Esselstyn, Jr., also one of the earliest pioneers of a plant-based diet has been recognized as one of the top doctors in the country in Steven Woodward Naifeh and Gregory White Smith's influential book *The Best Doctors in America*. He has undoubtedly been one of the most influential doctors with his benchmark, long-term nutritional research study, "A Strategy to Arrest and Reverse Coronary Artery Disease: A 5-Year Longitudinal Study of a Single Physician's Practice," which has continued on for decades more. In this study, he focused on a group of the sickest of heart patients who were not expected to live more than a few years. He used natural treatment modalities versus conventional medications and procedures to stop and reverse coronary artery heart disease. He published his findings in 1995 and again in 2014 when he reported the on-going experiences of the 198 participants.

Follow-up showed that of the 89 percent who followed through with the program, 99.4 percent avoided further major cardiac events. That study was reviewed beyond twenty years in his book *Prevent and Reverse Heart Disease*, making it one of the longest longitudinal studies of its type. Twenty-five years later, all but one of his patients were still living. The guidelines for these patients were easy. They could only eat whole plant food—no meat, dairy, oil, and minimal salt and sweeteners.

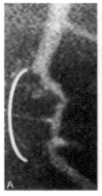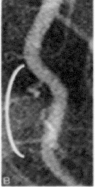

This image shows a coronary artery scan (angiogram) of people with significant heart disease before and after five-years on a whole food plant-based diet. As you can see, the one on the right is like that of a young healthy person with no vessel disease. Those who followed Dr. Esselstyn's program, maintained cholesterol levels below 150 mg/dl. They had no recurrent coronary events leading up to the twelve-month follow-up visit and 70 percent showed reversal of stenosis, which is the abnormal narrowing of a blood vessel. This same group of patients had more than forty-nine coronary events during the eight years prior to this study under the alternative recommended treatment modalities.

The original standard for controlling cholesterol levels has been set at 200 mg/dl, a number that, in 1989, many scientists on the Research Council on Diet and Health felt—and still feel—is too high. They believed that the target should have been set at 150 mg/dl, which has proven to be what it should have been in the first place. According to the long-running Framingham study, which has been instrumental in predicting people's risk for heart disease, 35 percent of ischemic heart disease occurs in patients with cholesterol levels between 150 and 200 mg/dl, and the average heart attack occurs at just slightly above 200 mg/dl (206 mg/dl).

Cholesterol-lowering medications targeted at keeping cholesterol levels below 200 mg/dl, an increase in exercise, and dietary modifications to keep fat intake at less than 30 percent have repeatedly shown to be ineffective at preventing heart disease. These measures have also been shown to provide only a temporary benefit leading to repeated interventional procedures like stent placement, artery clearing, bypass surgeries, and imminent premature mortality. The only method proven to reverse heart disease and extend the lives of heart disease patients is following a whole food plant-based diet. Looking at these images, even individuals who are untrained in identifying scan results can clearly see the significant improvement of the vessels on the right.

Dr. Esselstyn and his wife, Ann Crile Esselstyn, have followed a plant-based diet since 1984. Their daughter, Jane, has also been pivotal support in the kitchen. Anne and Jane have created an extremely focused, healthy, and obviously scientifically driven cookbook with Dr. Esselstyn's guidance. It is called *The Prevent and Reverse Heart Disease Cookbook.*

Their son Rip Esselstyn is a firefighter who identified the prevalence of heart disease and diabetes in fire stations around the country. He set out to teach his fellow firefighters how they could reverse disease as well. He has dedicated his life to changing how firefighters and the general public eats through speaking engagements, health training programs, plant-based food products, and his remarkable *Engine 2* cookbooks. His Engine 2 health food products are available at health-oriented stores like Whole Foods.

See Dr. Esselstyn's site at Dresselstyn.com to enjoy all the fantastic success stories of people whose lives have been saved and improved by his research. You will also see many inspiring videos online of his generous family, who have worked together on this mission to help people for free by offering cooking demonstrations, gardening tips, and furthering education on plant-based lifestyles.

Dr. Neal Barnard

Dr. Neal Barnard founded the Physicians Committee for Responsible Medicine (PCRM) in 1985 because he wanted to promote *preventive medicine* versus *reactive medicine*. According to Dr. Barnard, drinking just two glasses of cow milk a day increases human cancer risk by 60 percent, meat consumption is linked to a 28 percent increase, and the average Western diet, rich in processed and fast food, increases risk 200 percent. With meat and dairy specifically linked to increased cancer risk, Dr. Barnard says, giving up animal products is one of the best things a person can do to decrease their risk of developing cancer or experiencing cancer cell growth.

Dr. Barnard has authored many highly rated books, including *Foods That Cause You to Lose Weight I & II, Foods That Fight Pain, Turn off the Fat Genes, Breaking the Food Seduction, Dr. Neal Barnard's Program for Reversing Diabetes, Cookbook for Reversing Diabetes, The Cancer Survivor's Guide, and 21-Day Weight-Loss Kickstart.* He is also a worldwide speaker on the science of whole food plant-based dietary lifestyles and is very well versed in the differences between the digestive systems of omnivores (meat and plant eaters) and herbivores (plant eaters) at the most specialized physiological level. Science shows that humans were once herbivores but have adapted, to some extent, to have some omnivore characteristics.

Unfortunately, still today, we are not built to successfully digest meat, dairy, or fish without consequences. The protein and fat in this food wreak havoc on our bodies, causing about 90% percent of all the health problems plaguing America.

We share stunning similarities to herbivores in the design of our gastrointestinal system, which is very different from omnivores' systems in many ways. Herbivores share the presence of enzymes in their saliva, just as we do. These enzymes begin breaking down plant carbohydrates in our mouths during chewing and throughout digestion. Our front teeth are dull and slide over each other. Our molars are flat and wide. Our jaws move freely in all directions. Food is easily mashed and ground, helping to prevent chunks of food that cause choking. The length of our intestines is much longer in relation to our torsos. We have extensive, complex, striated linings in our intestines, where the exchange of nutrients occurs, allowing food to sit for extended amounts of time and excessive exogenous fat to build up.

Omnivores do not share these same characteristics. They lack the digestive enzymes for breaking down plant carbohydrates, their teeth surfaces are not nearly as smooth, their jaws are limited, and chunks of food are passed on to the stomach easily and quickly. Since omnivore and carnivore intestines are much shorter than herbivores' and the lining is smooth, fat passes through quickly.

Interestingly, humans who regularly consume meat and dairy products can easily develop cardiac disease and heart attacks, but most carnivores and omnivores do not.

Dr. Barnard is also very knowledgeable about the long history of various fad diets, including the ever-popular Atkins Diet. This diet promotes weight loss by allowing you to eat all the fat and protein you want and avoid carbohydrates, which goes against eating plant food. The Atkin's diet is a common discussion topic among nutrition scientists. Several scientists who speak at the *International Plant-Based Nutrition Healthcare Conference* have stated that the Atkins Diet has become one of the most health-damaging diets in history. Information found on Dr. Barnard's site at PCRM.org includes a National Institutes of Health study of more than half a million people, which showed that eating red and processed meat increases the risk of total mortality, cancer mortality, and cardiovascular disease mortality. Low-carb, animal-based diets such as Atkins are associated with early death. And research presented at the *American College of Cardiology's 68th Annual Scientific Session* found that low-carb diets increase the risk for atrial fibrillation, which is associated with a five-fold increased risk for stroke and may lead to heart failure. Low-carb diets have also been linked to increased colon cancer risk, the formation of kidney stones, kidney disease, and even osteoporosis."

He went on to say, "The weight loss you see in low-carb diets isn't all that much better than what you see in studies of low-fat, vegetarian diets." The Atkins Foundation asked Dr. Barnard to speak at their conference, and he states that he saw that as a sign that people are finally open to change.

The following chart shows some of the differences between species, food consumption, and digestion features.

Anatomical Feature	Carnivores	Omnivores	Herbivores	Humans
Anatomical Features of Carnivores, Omnivores, Hervibores, and Humans				
Incisors	Short, pointed, or sharp	Short, pointed, or sharp	Broad, flattened, or spade-shaped	Broad, flattened, or spade-shaped
Canines	Long, sharp, pointed and curved	Long, sharp, pointed and curved, or none (ex. chicken)	Dull, short, long, or none	Short and blunted
Molars	Sharp, jagged, blade-shaped, and/or flattened	Sharp, jagged, blade-shaped, and/or flattened	Flattened with cusps	Flattened with nodular cusps
Jaw	Unable to move jaw sideways to chew	Unable to move jaw sideways to chew	Able to move jaw sideways for grinding High chewing capacity	Able to move jaw sideways for grinding High chewing capacity
Colon	Simple and short	Simple and short	Long and complex	Long and complex
Nails	Sharp claws	Sharp claws	No sharp claws Flattened or blunt nails or hooves	No sharp claws Flattened or blunt nails
Intestinal Length & function	3 times the length of torso Smooth - allowing fats to pass through quickly	3-6 times the body length Smooth - allowing fats to pass through quickly	10-12 times body length Striated - fats remain longer, and are absorbed slowly	12 times length of torso Striated - fats remain longer, and are absorbed slowly
Saliva	No digestive enzymes: cannot detoxify Vitamin A	No digestive enzymes: cannot detoxify Vitamin A and unable to digest certain plants	Have carbohydarate digestive enzymes to detoxify Vitamin A and able to begin plant digestion orally & throughout	Have carbohydrate digestive enzymes to detoxify Vitamin A and able to begin plant digestion orally & throughout

The relatively short intestinal length in carnivores and omnivores, along with the relatively smooth interior surface, allows animal protein and fat to pass through quickly, whereas the longer striated intestines slow them down, causing a buildup in human intestines. You may never see true carnivores or omnivores with clogged arteries. You don't typically hear about pets having atherosclerosis, open-heart surgery, or stent placements.

Dr. Dean Ornish

Dr. Dean Ornish researched the impact of diet and stress levels on people with heart disease. The research, published in peer-reviewed journals, became the basis of his book *Program for Reversing Heart Disease*. The program combines diet, meditation, exercise, and support groups and became the first nonsurgical, nonpharmaceutical therapy for heart disease to qualify for insurance reimbursement, including Medicare. Dr. Ornish was a physician consultant to former President Bill Clinton after his cardiac bypass grafts became clogged. Clinton was encouraged to follow a mostly plant-based diet, and consequently, he lost a great deal of weight. Dr. Ornish has written many books, including *Dr. Dean Ornish's Program for Reversing Heart Disease*; *Eat More, Weigh Less*; *Every Day Cooking with Dr. Dean Ornish*; *Love & Survival: The Scientific Basis for the Healing Power of Intimacy*, *The Spectrum*, and *UnDo It!* with Anne Ornish. For a fascinating interview where Bill Clinton discusses how he lost weight on a plant-based diet, go to https://vimeo.com/155375404.

The research conducted over the last thirty-five years for Dr. Ornish's Program for Reversing Heart Disease has shown that a low-fat, whole-food plant-based diet approach can reverse heart disease and other chronic diseases. In Dr. Ornish's large-scale study with cardiac disease patients on a plant-based diet, 82 percent showed improved vessel stenosis at one year. Meanwhile, 91 percent had reduced or no chest pain without using lipid-lowering medications compared to a conventional care group with lipid-lowering meds and usual procedures who experienced increases in chest pain and higher cholesterol levels.

In Dr. Ornish's book *UnDo It*, his recommended diet and lifestyle program is a high-level type of vegetarian diet that can relieve the symptoms of heart disease. The diet has gained popularity in the last thirty years because participants lose more than twenty-four pounds on average, and most of them keep the weight off permanently, unlike most other diets and eliminates or reduces the risk factors of heart disease. The Ornish Diet's positive effects have been documented through research, which is why many doctors and health professionals prescribe it for their patients. The diet encourages people to eat all the beans, legumes, fruit, grains, and vegetables they need to feel full, and low to moderate amounts of low-fat dairy products. If that doesn't work to bring down your risk factors, you are encouraged to avoid all meat, oil, and sugar. Especially when followed at its highest level, this diet can reverse disease just as a Whole Food Plant-Based Diet does, but with the added emphasis of stress reduction, meditation, love, and support. Results vary from person to person, but people have lowered their body mass index by more than 10 percent, lowered their cholesterol by forty points, and lowered their systolic blood pressure by thirty-five points.

Thanks to scientists like Dr. Ornish and the others in this chapter, the world of nutritional science is becoming more accessible. Finally, programs are popping up all over the country that can help. Due to the popularity of Dr. Ornish's programs and the expense involved for coverage through Medicare, you must have some pretty serious underlying heart disease to be accepted. Call your hospital system or go online to see if his Nutrition as Medicine Lifestyle program has come to your area. If so, contact your doctor or call Dr. Ornish's center directly to see if you qualify.

Many doctors are not yet aware of the program or how it works. If you do not qualify, don't fret. You can do the program yourself by following the guidelines in this book and with the other resources referenced, along with ongoing monitoring by your physician. If you are ready for the challenge, you must be bold and convince your doctor that you are more interested in learning about health and nutrition for healing rather going the route of taking medications and impending procedures. Tell him or her that you want their assistance to help guide and monitor you on your new journey to health. It is not difficult for them to do a consult, order regular labs, and make sure you are on the right track. Our government and healthcare system are finally beginning to understand the huge benefit and cost savings this way of life brings.

If you live in a remote area, doctors can give you the support you need via telehealth appointments, and today you can order everything you need with regard to food items and resources online.

Fun Fact: I attended a conference here in Virginia Beach, Virginia to listen to two of my favorite local, well-respected doctors, Dr. Roshan Talreja and Dr. Deepak Talreja, both of them specialists in the fields of cardiology and internal medicine. Dr. Roshan Talreja recalled medical conferences about twenty years ago when Dr. Ornish came to speak. He stated, "During a conference for doctors back then, behind the scenes, they were saying that the way Dr. Ornish looked at 'Nutrition as Medicine' was crazy, but it turns out today that he was right all along."

Dr. Michael Klaper

Dr. Michael Klaper has been helping people reclaim their health through proper nutrition for more than forty years. He is well-known for explaining complex medical topics in plain, simple English and enjoys witnessing thousands of people worldwide accomplishing the reversal of chronic disease. He travels to medical schools around the country to teach young medical professionals the key role of diet as the cure for chronic illness by promoting plant-based nutrition as a part of the medical school curriculum for all healthcare professionals.

Some simple, well-known statements by Dr. Klaper are: "Meat protein leads to colon cancer, autoimmune diseases, and type 2 diabetes." "High protein diets are toxic to the kidneys and result in dialysis." "The keto diet after five days leads to acidosis and stress on your kidneys, causing bone and liver damage", not to mention kidney failure, and "Humans are carb-burning organisms. Our mitochondria burn glucose, not fat!"

Dr. Klaper and many of the other scientists in this book are not advocates of extended fasting. He believes that fasting is easily and best done on a daily basis on a plant-based diet by simply eating the last meal of the day around four or five p.m. The body only needs about thirteen hours to be in a state of ketosis, and "thirteen to fourteen hours is a perfect fasting period for cleansing the body of toxins on a daily basis." If you eat breakfast at about seven a.m., you will have fasted for fourteen or fifteen hours. Some people may need more extended fasting to reset their taste buds and microbiomes but require medical supervision. See his free videos at Doctorklaper.com.

In Closing

There you have it in a nutshell, so to speak—the star doctors who have blazed a trail for you and me to change the way we eat and reset our lives for the better. I encourage you to check out their websites, books, articles, and other material and expand your knowledge of their work. The extra knowledge you'll glean can only help you continue to improve your diet and your life.

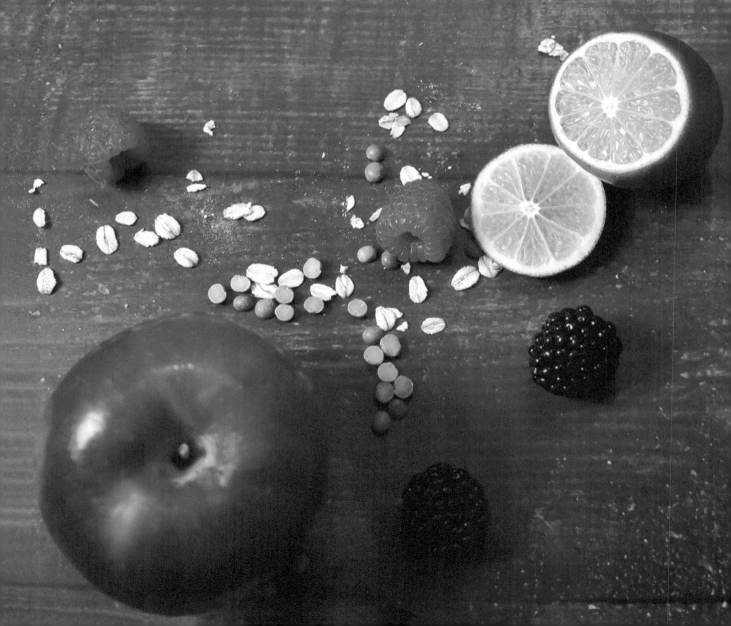

PART 3

The Whole Food Plant-Based Diet
For Specific Populations

CHAPTER 10

Pregnancy and the Whole Food Plant-Based Diet

Are you one of the many people who question whether it's safe for pregnant women to consume only whole plant-based food while pregnant? Put your worries to rest. Hands down, plant-based eating is absolutely better than the Standard American Diet for pregnant women, as it is for everyone else. The plant-based food a fetus gets from their mother nutritionally supplies them with everything they need and gives them the healthiest start to forever health when done right.

If you want further reassurance that a WFPBD is suitable for pregnant women, investigate to the American Dietetic Association, an organization with over 100,000 certified practitioners, as well as the British Dietetic Association and National Health Service. They state that plant-based eating is healthy and adequate for all persons, including pregnant and lactating women. They also note that plant-based diets followed correctly "reduce preeclampsia rates to 1 in 775 pregnancies versus the usual 1 in 25"[34].

So, if you're pregnant, don't let that stop you from considering adopting a whole food plant-based lifestyle. Of course, it is advised that you to consult with your doctor on your health needs during this time.

A WFPBD and Nutrition During Pregnancy

During pregnancy, a woman's nutrient needs increase. For example, she will require more protein, calcium, vitamin D, B12, iron, folate, omega fatty acids, iodine, and folic acid, even though her calorie needs will increase only modestly. Women don't need to pack on a lot of extra calories or protein during pregnancy because on a whole food plant-based diet they get all the nutrition they need without the unnecessary fat and calories of a SAD. An additional 340 calories are all that is necessary during their second trimester. And into the third trimester, they need only an additional 450 calories. There is no need for meat, fish, or dairy, but to be sure all nutrients are covered, prenatal vitamins are recommended by most obstetricians and pediatricians for those on both plant-based and animal-based diets, especially those who aren't sure they are consuming a good variety of healthy vegetables, fruits, legumes, grains, nuts, and seeds.

A pregnant woman who wants the best health for her baby will also limit or eliminate empty calories found in processed sugar, salt, and other processed food. Caffeinated coffee and alcohol in wine or beer should also be limited or eliminated during pregnancy. Any amount of caffeine or alcohol can affect a baby's metabolism and development. That said, some obstetricians make allowances for caffeine less than 200-300 mg per day and a half a glass of wine daily for those who feel it is too hard to abstain due to reasons given such as stress, anxiety, or fatigue. Better ways to manage all of these are activities like those mentioned in chapter 6, including yoga and meditation, maintaining regular exercise, going to bed earlier, increasing the amount of sleep you get, and eating well.

Your doctor can check your vitamin and nutrient levels in a simple blood test to ensure you are within an acceptable range for increased needs during pregnancy. Good news is if you follow the guidelines for a high-level whole food plant-based diet you can graze all day long and not worry about weight gain or associated health complications.

Now, let's take a more in-depth look at a pregnant woman's nutritional needs and how a WFPBD can satisfy them. Check vitamin/nutrient levels on prenatal vitamin labels and consult your obstetrician for further details.

Protein

A pregnant woman should aim for about 70 grams of protein per day during her second and third trimesters. It's easy to meet this requirement by eating a variety of plant-based food including lentils, quinoa, tempeh, tofu, whole grains, nuts, seeds, fruit, and vegetables. A day's menu could include oatmeal with fruit, walnuts, and crushed chia seeds or flaxseeds for breakfast; colorful vegetables and lentil soup and/or a hummus sandwich for lunch; quinoa, almond, and chickpea bowl with colorful vegetables or a salad with chickpeas for dinner; and a slice of whole-grain bread with peanut butter or sesame butter mixed with or sprinkled with flaxseed and fruit for a snack.

Calcium

The diet should include plenty of calcium-rich plant food during pregnancy, and the best sources are from chia seeds, flaxseeds, dark green leafy vegetables, figs, sunflower seeds, tahini, almond butter, and beans, including soy and tempeh. The Dietary Reference Intake level for calcium has been maintained for pregnant women at 1000 mg per day.

Vitamin D

The natural source of vitamin D-2 is made from plants like mushrooms when exposed to sunlight. Vitamin D-3 is made in the skin when exposed to sunlight and is the most readily absorbed form of Vitamin D. If one does not get regular sunlight, they can also get vitamin D-3 from supplements, which are generally made from sheep's lanolin/oil and added to food fortified with it like many brands of cereal and plant milk. Most prenatal vitamins contain 400 IU, but many obstetricians and nutritional experts recommend 2000 IUs during pregnancy.

Vitamin B12

Vitamin B12 is not found in most plant food, and it's difficult to acquire adequate amounts of it from both plant and nonplant food. To get enough of this vital nutrient, a pregnant woman should include a regular B12 supplement. She can consume plant-based forms of cheese, creamy dips, dressings, fortified soy milk, and cereal made with nutritional yeast as they usually contain plenty of B12 (check labels to be sure). This vitamin plays an essential role in the developing fetus and is also found in many multivitamins and prenatal vitamins. Most prenatal vitamins contain 10 mcg, and prenatal nutritional experts usually recommend up to 50 mcg daily or at least 2,000 mcg weekly.

Iron

Iron is abundant in plant-based diets. Legumes, dark leafy greens, dried fruit, blackstrap molasses, nuts, seeds, and whole-grain or fortified bread and cereal all contain iron. However, women in the second half of pregnancy sometimes need to take a supplement regardless of the type of diet they are on. Discuss iron supplements with your healthcare provider.

Folate (aka folic acid or Vitamin B9)

Folate is an integral part of proper brain development in babies. The baby's brain is rapidly developing in the first few weeks of pregnancy, and prenatal vitamins often contain sufficient amounts of folic acid. Plants like dark leafy greens, asparagus, broccoli, citrus fruit, beans, avocado, seeds, nuts, peas, and lentils contain plentiful amounts of folate as well. You can easily meet folate needs on a high-level plant-based diet. For those women on a SAD, the American College of Obstetricians and Gynecologists state that women of childbearing age should take 400 mcg of folate daily, and during pregnancy folate intake should be increased to 600 mcg of folic acid.

ALA, DHA, and EPA - Omega Fatty Acids

DHA and EPA, the omega fatty acids described in Chapter 3 are very important before getting pregnant, during pregnancy, and while breastfeeding. Studies have shown that some vegan moms without supplementation have significantly lower stores of DHA in their breastmilk compared to vegetarians and meat-eaters. Children who did not develop with adequate amounts of DHA were shown to be at increased risk for language development difficulties and visual acuity problems[35]. This is likely due to the fact that certain nutrients needed for the body to be able to convert ALA to DHA and EPA are not being consumed. This prompted the recommendation for preformed DHA and EPA supplementation of at least 250 mg per day[36, 37]. The bottom line is that ALA, EPA, and DHA can all be acquired through plant-based eating that includes nuts and seeds (walnuts, chia seeds, flaxseeds) combined with marine-sourced DHA/EPA (algae and seaweed) or an algae-derived omega supplement. It is better to get omega fatty acids from flaxseeds, chia seeds, and algae versus fish because of lead, mercury, DDTs, PCBs, and other pollutants[38]. These toxins can cause mental retardation and birth defects in children.

Iodine

Iodine is also best acquired from sea vegetables. During pregnancy, iodine is necessary for controlling blood pressure and preventing stunted growth and altered brain development of the fetus[22]. See the excellent video, *Supplements Before, During and After Pregnancy* at NutritionFacts.org. Most women don't get enough iodine during pregnancy, and only about half of prenatal multivitamins contain any iodine at all. The National Institutes of Health states that the RDA for US women who are pregnant, lactating, or even planning a pregnancy should be increased to 220 mcg of iodine per day and 290 mcg per day for breastfeeding[23]. Iodine needs have become an increased concern with any diet type due to the switchover to sea salt and kosher salt, which contain very little if any iodine at all. Varieties of seaweed like dulse, laver/nori, alaria, and wakame are the recommended sources. Kelp is another source that is very high in iodine and is not usually recommended unless you can limit kelp intake accordingly. Iodine needs can easily be met by adding a small amount of kelp powder or kelp flakes to a shaker of salt seasoning substitute to be kept on the table to add to food in place of salt. A pinch can be added to any of your meals or sprinkled on salads or in soups. You won't even taste it at the minuscule amount required. You can also eat seaweed instead if you prefer. Maine Coast Sea Vegetables is one of the producers found online.

Breastfeeding - Calories, and Protein

The guidelines for breastfeeding mothers are similar to those for pregnant women. Milk production requires even more calories than pregnancy, so a breastfeeding mother will need to boost her food intake up a bit. During the first six months of breastfeeding, she will need 500 calories more than before she became pregnant, and then this drops to 400 calories during the next six months of breastfeeding. Protein needs are the same as during the second and third trimesters of pregnancy (see "Protein" section earlier in this chapter for more details).

Alcohol and Pregnancy

Many doctors will say that it's okay to drink a small amount of alcohol while pregnant, but in 2005, the American College of Obstetricians and Gynecologists, the Centers for Disease Control and Prevention, the Surgeon General, and others in the medical community concluded that because "alcohol readily crosses the placenta and there is no known safe level of alcohol consumption during pregnancy, and alcohol is a known teratogen (an agent or factor that causes malformation of a fetus) that can impact fetal growth and development during all stages of pregnancy . . . all recommend complete abstinence during pregnancy"[39, 40].

It only makes sense that any interruption or slowing of metabolism during rapid growth periods, which alcohol can induce, is not optimal for producing the healthiest possible baby. Some people have referred to wine as a source to calm one's nerves during pregnancy, but there are healthier ways to manage that[41].

A Few More Words about Pregnancy and the WFPBD...

The WFPBD Is a Mood Stabilizer

Whole food plant-based eating is not only great for the mother and child's physical health, but it also stabilizes a pregnant woman's mood and sets the developing child up for better health down the road. Here's why: The body releases the hormone cortisol during times of physical and mental stress. Within a half-hour of consumption, a single meal high in animal protein releases nearly double the amount of cortisol in the blood as does a plant meal.

In pregnant women, high-meat, low-carb diets increase cortisol levels, leading to fetal exposure to cortisol. This affects the developing fetus, setting their automated stress hormone response, leading to higher cortisol levels for their entire life, with the potential for serious health consequences.

Dr. Neal Barnard is an excellent source for more information about plant-based diets as a healthful choice at every stage of life, including pregnancy and breastfeeding. You will find this and more on his site *Physicians Committee for Responsible Medicine* or *PCRM.org/good-nutrition/plant-based diets/pregnancy.*

Other popular resources for raising your family on a plant-based diet include Reed Mangels , Jack Norris, and Ginny Messina. They have written excellent books on this subject, and you can find them sharing information via video interviews online.

Dr. Mangels works for the Vegetarian Resource Group, a nonprofit organization that provides a wealth of information for families raising their children on vegetarian and vegan diets. The group can be found at www.vrg.org. The book *Simply Vegan* by Debra Wasserman and Reed Mangels is also a very popular resource.

Jack Norris and Ginny Messina are registered dieticians and coauthors of *Vegan for Life*. Ms. Messina learned a lot about veganism when she worked for Dr. Barnard's Physicians Committee for Responsible Medicine. Check out *www.VeganHealth.org* and *www.JackNorrisRD.com* for more information.

CHAPTER 11

Children and the Whole Food Plant-Based Diet

When my daughters were infants nearly thirty years ago, my husband and I introduced them to vegetables and fruit as soon as they were developmentally ready within pediatric recommendation guidelines. We blended everything we were eating to make homemade baby food for every meal. I was determined to ensure that our children ate only the best of the best we could offer. Despite our frequent military moves, I grew vegetables outdoors and indoors as much as possible. I was so serious about making my own baby food that my mother-in-law bought me an electric and battery-powered baby food masher so we wouldn't have to mash everything by hand.

Getting my children on the road to eating healthy early on has paid off. Today, my adult daughters try to maintain a healthy diet. My young son eats healthy fare, too. It has always been gratifying to receive compliments from friends and family about how well our children eat and how healthy and beautiful they are. It shocks people to see that my daughters, and now my son, would eat everything, even food such as spinach, onions, and peppers at such young ages. Frequently, they asked how in the world we made that happen.

Children are rapidly growing and require great amounts of healthy nutrients for proper development. It can be difficult to monitor them sometimes, especially when they are at the mercy of schools and other caregivers. Check the labels of any pre-packaged food they may eat and talk to your doctor about the best quality multivitamins and supplements. Do this to ensure your children are getting enough of the right nutrients on any diet. Place more emphasis on a variety of whole plant-based food and be especially focused on their intake of calcium, vitamin D, B12, zinc, iron, omegas, and iodine. Refer to vitamin and element charts for Dietary Reference Intakes at the
National Institutes of Health[1].

Start your children on whole plant-based food and give them the gift of a lifetime of health and happiness.

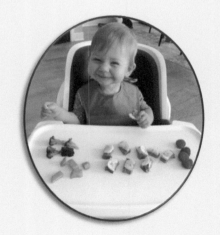

My advice: If all you do is feed your children what you eat, and what you eat is healthy, everything needed for a healthy, happy lifetime will easily fall into place. The "one bite" rule has always been a big one in our home—having our children take at least one bite of every food item on their plate each meal helps them adapt over time. Other successful tools are patience, love, reasoning, and food presentation with creative shapes, colors, and arrangements to make healthy eating fun. If you remember from earlier in the book, nature is on your side: Very young children and infants instinctively go for calorie-dense food. You might expect them to choose only sweet or colorful food, but studies show that they select green beans over melons and potatoes over peaches . . . that is until they are fed unnatural processed food like white sugar, white bread, cheese, candy, and fried food. So, try to avoid feeding them those things, or do so very seldomly and in very small amounts after they've had an appropriate nutritious meal.

My son is very involved in packing his lunchbox for school. An example of food he enjoys include whole grain spaghetti with homemade plant-based sauce and "parmesan cheese", cucumbers, carrots, blueberries, peanut butter mixed with crushed flaxseeds (containing omega oils), bananas on whole wheat bread, and homemade applesauce. He loves helping me make his lunches. We have a lot of fun trying to be creative with choosing various colors of food. Breakfast consists of whole grain cereal, nondairy milk, a daily vitamin, an algae omega supplement, and a daily or weekly B12 supplement. We make sure he gets outdoors in the sunshine to get the full natural benefits of vitamin D3, and in the winter, he gets about 800 mg of a Vitamin D supplement and he is a very healthy, strong, and brilliant boy.

Children: WFPBD

Many kids are picky eaters because they are creatures of habit and familiarity. Once they are accustomed to unhealthy food, they don't easily transition to healthy food and they are limited in their desire and ability to understand nutrition.

Children, Dairy, and Diabetes

We've already discussed how animal protein works with fat to cause atherosclerosis and overall heart disease in adults and children, but diabetes is yet another soaring concern for children. There are two genetic variants of cow's milk protein: A1 and A2 beta-casein. In experiments performed on children with diets containing A1 beta-casein from cow's milk, nearly half of them became diabetic, but studies showed low to no risk of diabetes in those who drank A2 beta-casein milk, which is now rarely found in the US. Additionally, it has been determined that children on nondairy diets and prolonged breastfed babies have a lower risk of developing type 1 diabetes. The standard Holstein cows common in the United States produce the A1 beta-casein protein which is believed to be a significant contributor to destroying the insulin-producing cells in children with type 1 diabetes[42]. Given this information, it is no wonder that diabetes was once unheard of, but now eight-year-olds are becoming diabetic at an increasing and alarming rate.

Excellent videos by Dr. Greger on this subject can be found online at NutritionFacts.org, including *Does Casein in Milk Trigger Type I Diabetes?*

Children and Heart Disease

As demonstrated in the study "Atherosclerotic Cardiovascular Disease Beginning in Childhood," data shows that children as young as three have exhibited fatty streaks in their vessels. Studies have also revealed fatty streaks or early cholesterol in fetuses, and clear evidence from autopsies demonstrates that nearly 100 percent of children on the SAD, at age ten, a fact previously mentioned in this book, have fatty cholesterol in their vessels[43]. Atherosclerosis begins in childhood as an accumulation of fatty streaks in the intima of the arteries. It may or may not progress to form plaques that undergo calcification, hemorrhage, rupture, and thrombosis[44].

Meanwhile, multiple studies have shown that the less fruit and veggies and the more meat and dairy kids eat, the higher their heart disease, cancer, and diabetes risk is overall.

Children and the WFPBD: The Parent and School Connection

As a mother of an elementary-school-age son and now as a grandmother, all of this information about the effect of dairy and meat on children really disturbs me, but it is a relief to know that such harmful conditions can be reversed with the right food in just a few weeks if done early enough and correctly. The problem is that schools don't offer all the necessary food options in the cafeteria, and many parents don't pack healthy meals in their children's lunchboxes.

My son attends a state-of-the-art public school that the city considers the best in offering everything, including healthy lunches. His school does a pretty good job as far as public schools go, but it is limited by nutrition education and what the government system provides. Children are strongly influenced by their peers who, for the most part, are eating school cafeteria lunches. Milk, meat, and cheese are still a big problem as there are no nondairy milk options offered at most schools. Public schools are still serving dairy milk, which has been proven to cause many diseases in children, including irritable bowel syndrome, obesity, lactose intolerance, fatty vessel streaks, and diabetes, as mentioned earlier. Sadly, as a former milk lover myself, finding out that even low-fat milk is unhealthy almost broke my heart.

Pizzas with dairy cheese, meatball subs, and macaroni with dairy cheese continue to be school favorites and as reported by my son and from what I've seen, the only other available healthy options are light green lettuce salads (not dark leafy greens) with croutons and occasionally a small amount of broccoli, green beans, or apples as a side.

The people making the lunch choices are well-intended, but again, most are misinformed. As for children who bring their meals to school, I find it interesting to join my son for lunch and see what his peers pull out from their lunchboxes. Over the years, I've noticed that some home lunches have evolved into more homemade stews, salads, fresh vegetables, grain bowls, fruit, nondairy milk, and less processed food. Sadly, obese children, children requiring heart medications, children with diabetes, and children with many other forms of inflammatory disease still have lunches loaded with processed sandwich meat, cheese, salami, cookies, Cheetos, and chips. They also have free rein to drink cow's milk and unnaturally flavored and processed sugar loaded drinks.

I see the impact of this not only in the lunchroom but also in the school nurses' office. I substitute as a nurse in school clinics and have witnessed a considerable increase in children with diabetes. It astonishes me how many kids are on insulin pumps. Many children come in first thing in the morning to test for high blood sugar levels after breakfast, and around lunchtime, we have to help them inject insulin to compensate for the high glycemic sugary meals they've eaten. They bring in their lunches, or what is left of them, and together we double-check what they consumed to make sure they have adjusted their insulin dosing properly. It really concerns me how many kids have blood sugar levels over 300, the number that signals that it's time to take more drastic measures. These children are at risk of emergent care and chronic disease progression, but so many of them seem, at times, to take pleasure in fighting their parents, nurses, and their doctor's orders to do further monitoring and adjustments of blood sugar levels.

More on the Importance of Getting Children on a WFPBD

Maybe what it will take to convince some parents to switch their children to a WFPBD is the horrific reality that could possibly await if they continue down the simple carbohydrate, processed, non-fiber food road they are on. I have seen that reality, and it is not pretty. I have worked with patients in the ICU due to diabetes complications, including amputations. I have taken care of patients at home with extreme wound care needs resulting from diabetes. Seeing firsthand the damage this disease can cause is shocking. Many of these patients are blind and/or have lost toes and sometimes entire legs. The rotting flesh wounds are some of the worst things I've ever witnessed in wound care. Hundreds of these poor souls live around us in their homes, unable to get out without assistance, or unwilling to. But children who have never seen this don't realize what sadness their future may hold. One of my daughters, who once thought she wanted to be a surgeon, traveled with me to do wound care on some of my patients and was horrified when she saw first-hand what I'm talking about. The good news is that these horrible diseases and their potential damage can be reversed or stabilized with a whole food plant-based diet.

We just need to get our kids started on a healthy lifestyle from the get-go.

CHAPTER 12

The Whole Food Plant-Based Diet, Disease, Disorders, and Surgery

Prevent or Reverse Disease with a WFPBD

It's not the easiest thing to contemplate, but the reality is that we were all born with a set of genes preprogrammed with susceptibility to certain diseases, a fact that should make each of us vigilant about what we choose to eat. Why? Consider this example as an explanation: Some of us may be more susceptible to carcinogens (cancer-causing agents) that activate particular cancers, but if we don't consume carcinogenic products, then we may never activate the gene(s). In other words, your disease, if you have one, may have been caused by the food you were raised on and continue to eat. Another example is the effect saturated fats and trans fats have on increasing the risk of developing Alzheimer's Disease. By avoiding cheese, ice cream, meat, milk, and egg products, people who have the gene for Alzheimer's reduce their risk of getting the disease by 80 percent. Yes, a whopping 80 percent!. As Dr. Greger's and many others' research has shown, it seems that what is bad for the heart is also bad for the brain. Oxidized cholesterol is a significant risk factor for Alzheimer's disease and results in hardening of the arteries in the brain, just as it does in our heart vessels. Oxidized LDL can cross the blood-brain barrier and has been shown to cause similar damage. Like Alzheimer's, many other diseases, of course, can be directly related to food consumption too. See Dr. Greger's video on Nutritionfacts.org: Oxidized Cholesterol as a Cause of Alzheimer's Disease.

Given that so many diseases may have a food-related cause, it's certainly worth our time to review our diets and consider overhauling them if they're putting us at risk of getting or remaining sick. So now we'll examine several diseases and disorders to see how and why adopting a WFPBD can cure, prevent, or diminish disease impact on you.

DIABETES - TREATING THE CAUSE NOT THE SYMPTOMS

You must have a stable foundation for everything, especially for your health. Doctors typically focus on treating the symptoms of diabetes with medications and don't normally focus on prevention, for reasons discussed earlier in Chapter 9. The reality is that diabetes often leads to blindness, peripheral vascular disease, and amputations. It also involves eating disorders, fatigue, mood disorders, sleep disorders, erectile dysfunction, etc. Often, patients are instructed to go on a low-calorie or low-carb diet, which for the general public is simply a way of starving and depriving themselves of the nutrients they need. They end up replacing good carbs with something equally as bad. Others are advised to eat a high-fat, low-carb diet, which worsens the problem. You see, there is a relatively new fact that many people are unaware of, and that is the involvement of fat in diabetes, which causes insulin resistance, inhibiting cell function, resulting in elevated sugar levels in the blood. The recommended diets for diabetics are very confusing. There isn't enough clarification about what a "low-carb diet" is and there isn't enough emphasis on how a diet rich in complex carbohydrates is beneficial. Rather than restricting carbs, people must be educated about replacing simple carbohydrates with complex carbohydrates, which are also known as whole plant food.

Contradictory to the advice given to patients in the past, the only way to get to the root cause of diabetes is to cut out saturated fat and processed trans fats and—this way, the insulin resistance in the cells is eliminated, allowing proper nutrients to be taken in by the cells to fuel the body and maximize function, thereby eliminating type 2 diabetes and controlling the progression of type 1 diabetes.

NOTE: Dr. Michael Greger and Dr. Neal Barnard have programs that will helps many long-time insulin-dependent type 2 diabetes patients get off of insulin in just two weeks. Find Dr. Greger's information in his books *How Not to Diet* and *How Not to Die*. Go to Dr. Barnard's site: The Plantrician Project, Journal of Disease Reversal and Prevention at https://ijdrp.org/index.php/ijdrp. Https://Diseasereversaldigest.com is another great source you can subscribe to.

Diabetes, Type 1 – Many Benefits of a WFPBD for this Population

Doctors don't know all the things that cause type 1 diabetes, but they do know that genetics play a role. Type 1 diabetes is an autoimmune disorder primarily caused by the destruction of insulin-producing cells in the pancreas. This usually means that patients are prescribed life-long insulin injections or have an insulin pump to treat it. But if caught early enough, testing shows that some patients may have some remaining function of their pancreatic cells. In these cases, the remaining function can be enhanced or sometimes even controlled with a proper diet. As noted in the previous chapter, some studies have shown a connection to A1 beta-casein found in cow's milk. Ingestion of animal products has been linked to the disease and viruses can direct your own immune system to attack your pancreatic cells. Though rare, signs of this type of damage can be tracked through antibody testing.

Over time, high glucose levels and cholesterol in your blood can harm the nerves and small blood vessels in your eyes, kidneys, and heart. These abnormal blood levels in diabetic patients can cause arteriosclerosis (hardening of the arteries) and atherosclerosis leading to heart attacks and strokes. People who have type 1 diabetes can live long, healthy lives. They just need to consume a healthy, fiber rich, plant-based diet, of complex dietary sugar, not simple sugar, minimizing or eliminating those food sources known to worsen the disease. Begin on a program specifically for diabetics to maximize your ability to live longer, happier, and with much less or no complications from this disease. See Dr. Greger's video: Type 1 Diabetes Treatment: A Plant-Based Diet.

Diabetes Type 1 - Whole Food Plant-Based Diet Benefits

* ***Insulin medication reduction.*** Studies show that insulin requirements decrease by about 35 percent in only four days, and over a six-month period, they can reduce by 45 percent.

* ***More predictable and easier to manage.*** When people with insulin-dependent diabetes follow a low-fat, low-sugar, plant-based diet, their blood glucose levels decrease and stabilize without the need to limit carbs and the feeling that they are starving themselves.

* ***Decreasing kidney disease risk.*** Even though you believe you can manage your blood glucose levels while consuming an animal-based diet, the increased protein of animal-based food and glucose level changes often lead to kidney disease. Blood vessels in the kidneys are damaged over time, and the kidneys have to work very hard to process the high levels of protein. Diabetes is the leading cause of chronic kidney disease, which can lead to dialysis and kidney failure.

* ***Eat as much as you want and still lose weight.*** If you replace all fat, which is 9 calories per gram, with complex plant food, which is 4 calories per gram, you can eat more than double what you usually eat, no longer starve yourself, and still lose weight.

* ***Reduced risk of diabetic neuropathies***. Blood flow increases throughout the body on a WFPBD by lowering the blood's viscosity or thickness and increasing cell function by eliminating fat and cholesterol blockages. This helps prevent and reverse diabetic neuropathic pain, numbness, and amputations.

* ***Increase in energy and happiness.*** Some of the most commonly reported experiences of diabetic patients on a WFPBD are increases in energy, happiness, improved digestion, and increased quality of sleep[45].

Diabetes Type 2 - Extra Caution with WFPB Dietary Changes

Insulin resistance is the cause of type 2 diabetes, the most common type of diabetes, and the drug most commonly used to treat it is metformin. Decades of studies show that in groups of healthy subjects placed on high-fat diets versus high-carbohydrate diets, the high-fat diet group would develop double the blood sugar levels. Despite this fact, there was a widespread belief for a long time that increased consumption of sugar and carbs was causing diabetes due to the elevation of sugar in the blood. However, in 2006, exhaustive studies conducted by Japanese scientists showed that diabetes is caused by insulin blockage by intramyocellular lipids (fat in the muscle cells). *Insulin normally acts as a key to open a cell for allowing sugar to enter and be used to produce energy, but this fat layer blocks that process, and sugar levels elevate in the blood instead. The type of fat that causes this is found mostly in saturated fat from meat, dairy, and eggs.* The unsaturated fat found in whole plant food like almonds, nuts, and avocados helps to reverse the problem.

Many people don't realize that type 2 diabetes can actually be reversed in a matter of days to a couple of weeks[46-49]. Patients typically are unwilling or think they cannot change their diet and lifestyle to reach this goal. Those who overcome these barriers and decide they want to pursue a plant-based diet should have their blood sugar levels closely monitored while doing so. For those who have difficulties reaching this goal with their current doctor, a great online reference is www.PlantricianProject.org. This is a resource for finding a plant-based doctor in or near your area. It is a relatively new platform growing in populated areas but may take more time to reach the more rural communities.

A great online video source is Dr. Neal Barnard's *How to Reverse Diabetes in 3 Steps*, which can be found at https://youtu.be/SuwR46p7wrA.

Celiac Disease and Gluten Sensitivities, Reversing Inflammatory Diseases

Celiac disease is an autoimmune disorder that attacks the small intestines. It affects about one percent of the world's population. About 40 percent have the genetic predisposition but don't have celiac disease symptoms, and only 1 percent of those with symptoms have the genetic component of the actual disease. There is a one in ten chance of having celiac disease if it is in your family's health history. The only current treatment for *actual* celiac disease is a strict, gluten-free diet.

Gluten is an insoluble protein made up of gliadin and glutenin proteins found in wheat, rye, and barley. It is the elastic chewiness in dough. Classic symptoms of celiac disease in children are bloating, diarrhea, abdominal pain, and weight loss. Adults are less likely to experience the diarrhea component and more likely to have strange symptoms like anemia, fatigue, and joint pain. Gliadin can trigger the attack of an autoimmune response, damaging the lining of the small intestines, resulting in malabsorption and nutrition problems. An intestinal biopsy is a conclusive test to determine celiac disease.

Many people with the same symptoms as those with celiac disease don't have the genetic component. There is also a condition known as nonceliac wheat or gluten sensitivity without celiac disease or wheat allergies.

In summary, one percent of the population tested actually tests positive for celiac disease, 1 percent tests positive for wheat sensitivities, and 2 percent has nonceliac gluten sensitivities, which is a total of only 4 percent of the population Nonceliac gluten and wheat sensitivities testing ruled out millions of people with symptoms, and only about 13 percent of them said they felt better after removing gluten from their diets, yet many stores have gone to extremes to carry gluten-free products and replace nutrient rich whole grains.

People are quick to cut out wheat products, which are typically very healthy, and they don't cut out bulgur wheat or wheat berries to determine if wheat is, in fact, the culprit. They cut out food like muffins, cakes, and other items containing all kinds of other possible allergens. *People tend to add more animal products when they remove wheat from their diets, resulting in the enhancement of other potential diseases. A better course of action is to get tested to see what the problem really is.* There is a 1 in 10,000 chance that a person with irritable bowel symptoms would be diagnosed with celiac disease[50].

Wheat has many significant health benefits if you don't have celiac disease as it is rich in iron, B vitamins, thiamin, riboflavin, folate, niacin, folic acid, and of course, fiber. There are many whole grain alternatives to those with gluten sensitivities, including gluten-free quinoa, buckwheat, brown rice, wild rice, oats, amaranth, millet, teff, corn, and sorghum, just to name a few. I will go into more detail on these and more later in the book. Also, for more information about gluten, check out *The Gluten Manifesto: Everything You Need to Know About Gluten*, accessible online and at PCRM.org, Physicians Committee for Responsible Medicine[51, 52].

CANCER

Stomach or Gastric Cancers

Salt has been implicated as the number one cause of stomach cancer. Meanwhile, studies show that curcumin from turmeric, garlic, and capsaicin from red chili peppers may inhibit the proliferation of human stomach cancer cells[53]. Saffron and cardamom are also known to be beneficial in reducing stomach cancer risk—all great spice options that can be used in everyday meal planning.

Kidney Cancer

Too much protein causes a great amount of stress on the kidneys. Once protein needs are met, the body must excrete the remainder. Dr. John A. McDougall, one of the most highly regarded doctors in studies on kidney cancer states, "For the past sixty years, doctors and patients should have known that the primary focus of attention for the preservation of the kidneys should be diet."

Studies have shown that as much as 25 to 50 percent of functional kidney capacity is destroyed after seven to eight decades of eating the typical protein-rich, animal-based Western Standard American diet. We've already seen that if we eat enough plant food, we will get enough protein. The human body needs less than 5 percent of its calories from protein to build all cell structures, enzymes, and hormones. The American Heart Association lowered its recommendations for a heart-healthy diet to include no more than 5 to 6 percent of total calories from saturated fat, which is just the amount found naturally in a WFPB diet.

Today, the many meat replacement products in stores contain isolated soy protein, comprising 35 percent or more protein content of total calories. As mentioned previously, ISPs are potentially harmful to the kidneys and increase cancer risk. They are found in many "plant-based" or "vegan" burgers, hot dogs, luncheon meats, sausages, protein shakes, protein bars, powders, and cheeses; but again, keep in mind that ISPs are not considered "whole" plant food when consumed in a concentrated form, so be sure to check the nutrition labels on products before overindulging.

Herbs and Spices for Prevention, Treatment of Cancers

Throughout history, several herbs and spices have been used as medicinal plants to treat various disease and provide a lot of beneficial health effects. For example, studies have shown that some antioxidants from herbs and spices like curcumin from turmeric, eugenol from cloves, and capsaicin from red peppers, have potent antioxidant and anti-inflammatory properties[53].

The following information was obtained primarily from the US National Library of Medicine, National Institutes of Health (a worldwide accessible studies database) in a comprehensive study called *Nutrients*. The study results are a combination of testing on humans and lab specimens. Countless information exists on pathways of effectiveness on cancer prevention and cancer treatment. We'll break this down further to see which herbs and spices have been linked to reducing the risk and progression of specific types of cancer.

HERBS AND SPICES THAT GENERALLY HELP HEAL AND RELIEVE DISCOMFORT	
Cardamom	Fights inflammation and soothes an upset stomach.
Chili Peppers	Contains capsaicin, which boosts metabolism and helps keep blood vessels healthy.
Cinnamon	Helps prevent and reduce inflammation, is a flavonoid-rich antioxidant that fights free radicals and bacteria, and helps control blood sugar.
Cocoa	Helps lower cholesterol levels, reduce blood pressure, and is full of antioxidants for fighting toxins and free radicals.
Coriander	Contains an abundance of linalool, a naturally occurring seed with anticancer effects.
Cumin	Rich in iron and antioxidants, promotes digestion, reduces foodborne infections, improves blood sugar levels, lowers cholesterol, and may promote weight loss.
Garlic	Helps reduce heart disease risk by lowering cholesterol and lowering high blood pressure.
Ginger	Soothes upset stomach, eases nausea, is anti-inflammatory, and contains antioxidants that help prevent cancer.
Parsley	Rich in flavonoids that help prevent cancer, reduce tumor size, and lower blood sugar levels.
Rosemary	Rich in antioxidants, prevents cell damage and has shown preventive effects for cardiovascular disease, diabetes, and various solid cancers; Smelling it may help boost memory.
Turmeric	Excellent source of curcumin, an antioxidant that reduces inflammation, helps alleviate pain, and may help prevent or slow Alzheimer's disease

Specific Cancer Types and Potentially Beneficial Herbs and Spices
(Reminder: consult your oncologist/physician before making any changes to your current diet)

LUNGS: Curcumin found in turmeric, black cumin, ginger, garlic, saffron, capsaicin found in red chili peppers.

LIVER: Curcumin, black cumin, rosemary, clove, galangal.

BREAST: Curcumin, black cumin, ginger, garlic, saffron, black pepper, red chili pepper/capsaicin, rosemary, clove, coriander/cilantro, cocoa, green tea, and small amounts of extra virgin olive oil may help kill some breast cancer cells. Also, fiber helps remove excess hormones, which reduces the risk of breast and ovarian cancer.

COLORECTAL: Curcumin, black cumin, ginger, garlic, onion, scallions, saffron, black pepper, red chili-pepper capsaicin, rosemary, clove, galangal, cinnamon, oregano, and green tea. Also, vegetables such as fava beans, purple potatoes, peanuts, onions, and tomatoes help kill and slow colon cancer cells. Those who regularly consumed at least two one-ounce servings of nuts each week demonstrated a 46 percent improvement in overall survival[53].

CERVIX: Curcumin, black cumin, and cloves .

PROSTATE: Curcumin, ginger, saffron, black pepper, red chili pepper capsaicin, rosemary, thyme, and capers.

Managing Side Effects and Treatment of Cancer

Herbs and spices do more than fight cancer and inflammatory diseases. Many are useful for reducing side effects and treating chemotherapy-induced indigestion, nausea, vomiting, and the metallic taste cancer patients commonly experience.

Ginger, garlic, turmeric, and organic ginger tea were shown to reduce cancer treatment side effects. During periods of nausea, it is advisable to eat bland food. Avoid hot, spicy, sour, and acidic food, snack throughout the day on healthy sources, and plan to eat five or more times per day if possible.

Ginger possesses antioxidant, anti-inflammatory, antifungal, antimycobacterial, and anticarcinogenic properties. A clinical trial showed that inhaled ginger aromatherapy might be a complementary therapy for chemotherapy-induced nausea and vomiting.

Curcumin also augments chemotherapy, allowing higher doses and protecting patients from toxic side effects like chemotherapy-induced indigestion, nausea, vomiting, and metallic taste.

Work closely with your medical team to determine which food or nutrients are appropriate for your individual plan of care.

Cancer-Fighting Food

Your plate should always be colorful. If it is limited to only brown, white, or yellow, you are missing out on essential antioxidants and phytonutrients that are vital in fighting cancer. Top anticancer vegetables are broccoli, cauliflower, Brussel sprouts, kale, red cabbage, spinach, beetroot, purple potatoes, tomatoes, and cocoa powder. Fermented soy products, watermelon, grapefruit, kiwifruit, papaya, cranberries, pomegranates, figs, strawberries, raspberries, blueberries, ginger, walnuts, organic ginger tea, and green tea are also helpful in stopping the spread of cancer and reducing the size of cancerous tumors. When preparing food, choose baking, roasting, steaming, or boiling instead of chargrilling or frying in oil.

Wine is sometimes recommended by doctors for people who have thickened blood from saturated fat and for "reducing anxiety". Alcohol, in any form, increases the risk of cancer. Don't be confused by wine being a "beneficial fruit" when it comes to cancer. It is harmful to the human liver and does, in fact, hasten cancer progression. Additionally, wine and other alcoholic drinks are processed, which means they do not fit the healthy criteria of a whole food plant-based diet, but whole grapes, especially darker grapes, on the other hand, do, and they are loaded with cancer-fighting antioxidants.

According to studies performed by Vincenzo Bagnardi, Ms.C., Marta Blangiardo, Ms.C., Carlo La Vecchia, M.D., and Giovanni Corrao, Ph.D., "Greater alcohol consumption was associated with a greater increase in cancer risk and most strongly increased the risk for cancers of the oral cavity, pharynx, esophagus, and larynx for the highest alcohol consumption. Appreciably smaller, although still statistically significant, are increases in risk for cancers of the stomach, colon, rectum, liver, female breast, and ovaries. For all types of cancer, significant increases in risk existed even at the lowest consumption level studied at two standard drinks per day"[53, 54].

Alcohol also slows body processes or metabolism for seventy-two hours and though it may help you fall asleep, it interferes with sleep cycles, making you tired the following day[55]. Consuming alcohol can result in poor food choices, causes unhealthy cravings just before or during sleep times, and lead to worsened anxiety.

SURGERIES, AND HEALING ON A WFPBD

Before we wrap up and head to the next chapter, I want to take a few minutes to share my personal discovery of how following a plant-based diet can make even a major surgery a much less worrisome experience.

A few years ago, when I had to undergo a pretty major surgery myself, I selected a doctor who was considered the best in our area. His entire practice thrives on an insistence that his patients follow a WFPBD for several weeks pre-and post-surgery. When I walked in the door and his staff began teaching me the diet requirements, I realized I had entered what could be described as, for me, a tiny utopian world. I felt right at home. Four weeks before surgery, his staff placed me on a specific nutritional program. I was about five foot two and 128 pounds. This program included a focus on getting most of my protein from beans, legumes, greens, and other vegetables. Their preference for an avoidance of all meat and dairy, with the exception of one egg and a tiny amount of white broiled chicken or salmon once a week was made clear. They urged heavy emphasis of spinach, kale, beans, whole grains, and pineapple for healing, along with a daily vitamin they created and sell worldwide.

Their expectation was that I continue this diet for at least four weeks following surgery. Though I knew a lot about the WFPBD tenets prior to selecting this doctor and his staff, I was not as fully engaged in it.

This was the phase in my family's life where I was still struggling to get my husband and son to commit to a whole food plant-based plan. We kept eggs, chicken, and other risky food in the fridge. As for myself, I was consuming about two or 3 eggs per week, salmon one or two times a month, and using small amounts of olive oil. I thought that was sufficient for me, though my primary care doctor was still lecturing me about my total cholesterol level which was difficult to keep under 200. So I chose to prepare for surgery by following this doctor's WFPBD and besting him one by actually doing the stricter version of the regimen. This involved cutting out the oils, fish, eggs, and chicken. After two weeks of following this plan, I had lost nearly ten pounds and felt amazing in the time leading up to my surgery. During the surgery, the anesthesiologist only had to use very minimal anesthesia to sedate me, and post-surgery recovery was unbelievably easy. I needed minimal pain medication after the surgery, using only Tylenol for a very short time, which I believe had a lot to with my body's enhanced sensitivity and ability to identify potential threats and heal better. I was up and eager to return to my regular routine within a couple of days—no drains required, minimal swelling or redness, rapid healing, very little bruising, lots of energy, and great strength. I was delighted with the whole process.

Shortly after that surgery, I seriously injured my shoulder when a bone deformity led to a significant tear in my labrum, causing my shoulder to become frozen. Preparation for this new surgery centered upon a continued focus on my new strict diet. I was confident that I would have another very easy surgery and recovery, similar to my previous experience. Many others who had gone through a torn labrum and frozen shoulder surgery warned me about the amount of pain, stiffness, swelling, refreezing, rehab torture, etc., I would experience. In the two months leading up to this surgery, as I was unable to do my usual workouts due to the injury, I focused on busy work to distract myself with continued and deeper plant-based research.

Following the surgery, I continued on a WFPBD. My weight further dropped to a low of about 112 pounds, a weight I had not seen since my twenties, all without regular exercise over these months. I do not recommend skipping workouts however, as we all know how important they are, but I was really enjoying my new skinny self. Not exercising further confirmed how much my diet contributed to my new low weight. It was amazing how easy it was to stay thin, something that was never easy for me previously. All earlier diets required significant effort and constant vigilance to restrict calories and to keep myself from eating.

I had the same experience with this surgery, pre, and post, that I had with the previous one: very little anesthesia for the procedure and rapid weaning from narcotics to over-the-counter anti-inflammatory meds for the therapy sessions. The day immediately following my surgery, I had my first physical therapy session, and I was walking around visiting some of my patients in the hospital. People were amazed that I was so happy and feeling incredible. Today, I have full function of my shoulder and no problems whatsoever.

So wouldn't you know, I have the whole food plant-based diet to thank for that. My fantastic surgeons and their staff deserve a lot of credit as well, of course.

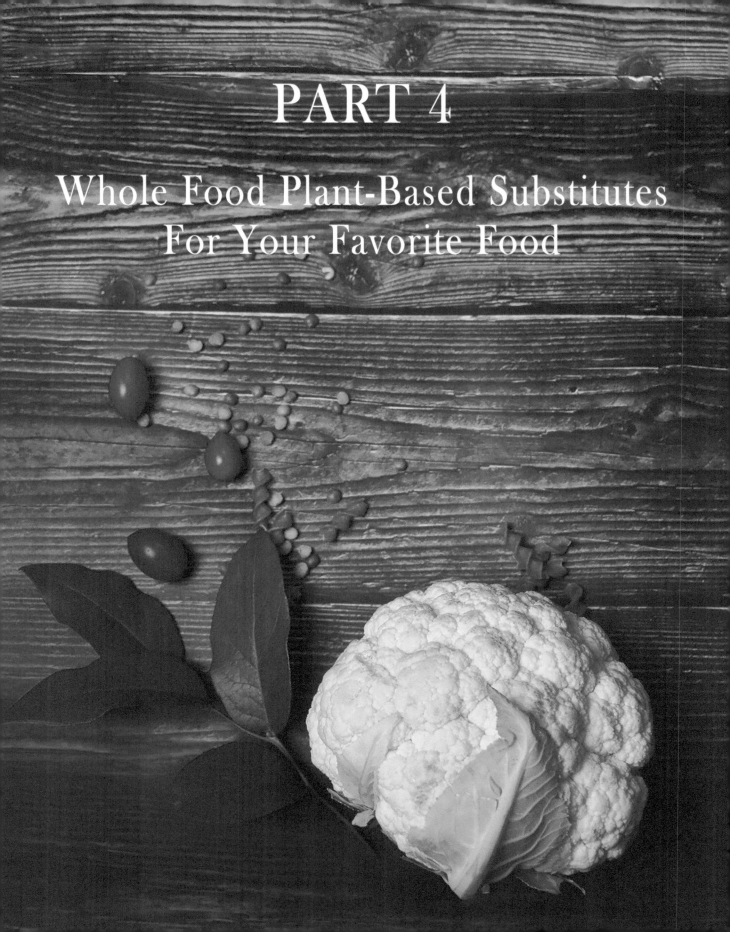

PART 4

Whole Food Plant-Based Substitutes For Your Favorite Food

CHAPTER 13

Healthy Substitutions for Everything

We often fear switching to a healthier diet because we take comfort in familiarity. It is difficult to give up the food we have spent our whole life eating. But take heart—many of the most difficult things to give up are things it is not necessary to actually give up! Instead, there are great replacements for nearly every favorite allowing the preparation of comparable dishes. Many of the substitutions I tout in this book come from experimentation with my family, replacing ingredients from family recipes as well as from the scientists and their families who are 100 percent whole food plant-based consumers.

Other sources include the Internet—with a plethora of risky recipe recreations that my family endured during our experimentation phase—as well as Blue Zone pioneers, others who have lived on plant-based, vegan, and vegetarian diets for decades, and cancer, diabetes, and cardiac support groups.

Before we look at all the great substitutions, however, I want to share with you how I learned to appreciate an abundance of fresh fruit and vegetables, ingredients you'll use often as you convert your favorite dishes to whole food plant-based creations. I came upon this love of this wonderful food earnestly.

It All Started in My Youth

I grew up in a typical family with three sisters, some animals, and an amazing garden, and I spent a lot of time helping my father tend to the garden and animals. My parents are very family-oriented, incredibly kind, welcoming, and very loving. They raised us on the healthiest food they could provide, often fresh from the garden. Rarely did we have to go to the local grocery store as our garden was an incredible bounty in itself. When visitors first arrived at our home, they usually wanted to tour the gardens and graze on our beautiful and delicious fruits and vegetables. It was amazing what we could do with a tiny piece of land.

My dad was always so happy to share his gardening methods with others and give out bags and bushels of everything he grew. Every year, out of our small garden, we would harvest bushels and bushels of tomatoes, onions, green peppers, beets, green beans, yellow beans, lima beans, cabbage, carrots, cauliflower, broccoli, peas, potatoes, peanuts, radishes, Brussel sprouts, asparagus, cucumbers, spinach, lettuce, turnips, strawberries, blueberries, blackberries, raspberries, golden raspberries, pears, peaches, apples . . . Shall I go on?

Some of the most interesting things my father has done are growing shiitake mushrooms and tending honeybee hives. The mushroom growing process fascinated me as he drilled holes in oak logs where he placed spores, kept them shaded, wet, and regularly rotated, tapping them to trigger growth. While wearing a bee suit with a smoker in hand to calm the bees, he paid particular attention to the quality of everything, including his honey, making sure it was pure, providing the bees plenty of fruit tree flower options and clover. My parents wanted nothing but the best food to raise their children on and were very self-reliant. They taught us everything we would need to know about gardening.

In addition to maintaining the garden, Dad was particular about the meat he provided for us. He has always been a hunter, bringing home geese, ducks, deer, rabbits, quail, and turkey. We rarely ate store-bought red meat, because even then, my parents considered it unhealthy. They thought wild-caught meat was healthy. Interestingly, we always had about a hundred or so rabbits that were our staple "protein." People often asked how it tasted and, the family joke was, "it tastes like watery chicken."

My mom was always a wonderful cook, and it was her mission to make sure we enjoyed the "healthy" food they provided.

Mom did a great job disguising the taste, but to be honest, I was never a big fan of any of the meat, and neither were my sisters. I would eat a tiny amount to try not to offend my parents and "get my protein." Back then, we believed that protein only came from meat. Our family drank store-bought milk and ate store-bought cheese and eggs. My happy place, however, was in the garden, grazing on fruit and vegetables. My sisters and I recall eating delicious fruit, entire green peppers, and onions while standing in the middle of the wonderful gardens.

My mom's goals were to disguise the gamey taste of our animal sourced "protein" and dad even created his version of barbecue deer meat that actually is quite delicious and indistinguishable from cow beef. Though I very much appreciate all the gifts my parents offered as I grew, when I was older and then began having a family of my own, I made many changes from old family dishes and now create new ones from the gardens that I maintain, both indoors and outdoors. Thanks to them.

You can see from my story that I grew up eating a Western diet that included meat, eggs, and dairy. My deep love of fruits and vegetables, food choices that are not typically "Western", is a direct result of the exposure to them by my parents. We were not aware back then that our recipes contained dietary health risks. As scientific and nutritional advances were made, I learned more about healthier eating and naturally gravitated toward learning how to concoct some of the tastiest whole food plant-based offerings.

Let's get ready to learn a bit more about the benefits of the healthiest ingredients and look at how you can swap them in, from fruits and vegetables, nuts, seeds, herbs, spices and more, to make your favorite meals whole food plant-based approved!

ALLERGIES AND PLANT-BASED EATING

If you have a food allergy, it is okay. You still have endless options for a healthy and delicious plant-based lifestyle. You can convert virtually every recipe with plant-based nonallergy options. It is essential to consult with your doctor before making any dietary changes if you have any health condition, questions, or concerns.

Nut Allergy Replacement Food Options

Interestingly, peanuts are classified as grain legumes, and more specifically, they are members of the bean and pea family and not actually considered a nut. Many people with peanut allergies are not allergic to other nuts. Have your doctor confirm your nut sensitivities before adding or leaving out certain types of nuts and legumes from your diet. Various options can be used as plant-based alternatives for people who are allergic to nuts.

Cashews are commonly used in many plant-based recipes because when blended, they provide a very creamy taste and texture and a subtle sweetness similar to some dairy cheeses, sauces, and creams, but for nut allergies, seeds are a great alternative. Seeds are a great substitute for nuts because they provide similar taste and often equally significant nutritional health benefits. Hemp seed butter and pumpkin seed butter are probably the closest alternatives in flavor and creaminess to cashews in making cheese and creams, though a downside of pumpkin seeds might be the green color. Sesame seed butter (tahini) and sunflower seed (SunButter), though very slightly bitter, are other delicious nut replacement options.

You can find seed butter in most stores or you can make your own by blending them for about ten minutes. Just get past the point where it is a paste in your blender. It's a fun experiment. Among other replacement options for making cheese and creams are cauliflower, white beans, white potatoes, and tofu. Nutritional yeast adds a delicious cheese flavor with a hint of hearty nuttiness and many more healthy nutrients. We will go into more detail on plant-based diets and allergies later in the book.

Next, we will jump right into other commonly requested information about food substitutions for which we all have been told to reduce or eliminate . . . for good reasons.

BAKING/COOKING SUBSTITUTIONS

NO SOS - SALT, OIL, SUGAR

Those who understand the benefits of healthy whole plant-based food and experience the amazing results do make significant changes, often saying goodbye to processed selections of salt, oil, and sugar. You too can replace these with healthier ingredients that you will grow to love. In a few weeks, you won't miss them, you will feel energized, the pounds will melt away, and many other great things will happen, resulting in a younger, stronger, and healthier you.

SUBSTITUTING SALT

As previously mentioned, salt is the number one cause of stomach cancer. Considerable evidence shows that it is also a significant cause of hypertension. It is a prevalent ingredient in processed food, packaged food, meat, and dairy. Many doctors believe that the primary cause of high blood pressure in patients who report that they control their sodium intake is referred to as essential hypertension. Essential Hypertension is documented in the medical textbooks as having an idiopathic (or unknown) cause. There is some assumption that there may be a genetic correlation in some cases, but tests would need to be done to determine that. What do doctors do when patients tell them they have controlled their salt intake, but their blood pressure is still high? They prescribe medications to bring their blood pressure down. There are several problems with that assumption and plan of care. One, studies have shown that identical twins are not identical at all when it comes to hypertension. When one twin is hypertensive, the other twin is hypertensive only 44 percent of the time. Two, in other countries where people eat naturally grown plant food without any added salt, there is no evidence of hypertension[56]. Yet another clear piece of evidence is that hypertension has rapidly increased in prevalence along with worldwide epidemics of obesity and diabetes rates over the last 100 years[57]. And both of these are significantly associated with...that's right! Drumroll please...Saturated fat, processed food, and consumption of protein and salt found in animal products. When hypertensive patients are put on diets that are very low in salt, such as a rice and fruit diet, their blood pressure falls toward normal levels[58]. Renal injury becomes the most likely mechanism of irreversible hypertension, and two of the key initiators are endothelial or vessel wall lining dysfunction and a hyperactive sympathetic nervous system, both of which can easily be related to what we eat. As noted earlier, it is believed that soy counteracts the damaging effects of salt, so let's review some of the ways soy can be used to help lessen these damages.

Soy Sauce, Bragg Liquid Aminos, and Tamari

Soy sauce, Bragg Liquid Aminos (non-GMO), or tamari (gluten/wheat-free) are derived from soybeans, an excellent protein source often used as a salt replacement. Keep in mind that even low-sodium soy sauce is high in sodium, though it's much lower in sodium than table salt. It measures at about 300 mg per teaspoon compared to salt at 2325 mg per teaspoon. A huge difference as you can see! It is commonly used in broths, gravies, salad dressings, chilies, curries, stews, marinades, peanut sauce, sautéing veggies, and more. Soy sauce is ubiquitous in Asian dishes. Japanese monks invented it to add a savory umami flavor (commonly pleasing taste perception) to vegetarian food. It tends to be saltier tasting than miso and lacks miso's creaminess. Bragg Liquid Aminos is derived from soybeans and is similar to soy sauce but is certified non-GMO and does not typically contain MSG. Tamari is a premium soy sauce made from more soybeans and has deep flavor than ordinary soy sauce.

Miso Paste

Also called bean paste, miso is made from fermented soy and grains like rice and barley. It comes in various flavors, textures, and colors. The whiter varieties are usually made with rice and are typically sweeter, milder, and used in salad dressings and sauces. The darker and redder varieties are usually made from soybeans, are saltier, and are mainly used to make broths. Miso has a salty, earthy, "savory" umami flavor, meaning it is a very appealing flavor that can taste salty, sweet, sour, and bitter. Miso can serve as a substitute for both salt and soy sauce and does not usually contain monosodium glutamate (MSG) or added processed sugars commonly found in store-bought products. As stated earlier, soy can help counter the harmful effects of salt/sodium on the vessels that cause hypertension and stomach cancer.

To make a quick vegetable broth, add 1 tablespoon miso paste (equal to about 1/4 or 1/2 teaspoon salt) to a cup of water. Darker miso, which usually contains the most sodium, has about 245 mg of sodium compared to table salt which has about 2,325 mg per teaspoon. That is a huge difference! The RDA limit for sodium is 2,300 mg per day (**NOTE:** This limit is believed to be too high, so The American Heart Association is working toward setting a standard sodium limit of 1,500 mg per day. Many medical professionals tell heart patients to avoid all added salt and avoid processed foods, but hypertension has continued to be a significant issue even with those rules. Miso can be used to flavor many things, like gravy, soup, stew, stir-fried vegetables, dressing, and mashed potatoes. As with sodium or salt, use it very conservatively. Miso paste is easier to use if it is diluted in an equal amount of warm water and stirred until smooth creating a *slurry*. When cooking with miso, try to add it last because boiling can destroy its beneficial enzymes, which boost your immune system and help feed the "good" microbes in your gut. Often in the stores, you can find miso in the refrigerator near the tofu or tempeh, in the international food section, or near the natural peanut butter in the organic or vegan food section.

Natural Salt, Soy Beans, and Soy Powder

Another option that I personally have made at home and prefer to use when working with dry recipe ingredients is soy powder made from soybeans. It is very handy to include in salt seasoning replacements and other homemade spices for helping to ensure you get the benefits of soy. You can find the recipe for *Soy Powder* in the second half of this book.

An interesting thing I've personally discovered about salt is how much better my eyes and body feel since I've significantly reduced my salt intake. I do this by not only incorporating soy into my diet, but by eating at home as often as possible and by replacing salt with herbs, spices and alternative flavor sources such as vinegar, lemon, and lime. Apparently, I sleep with my eyes open and, as a result, I used to wake up with terribly dry, puffy eyes in the middle of the night. It was so bad that I could hardly see to find my eye drops. Since then, I've switched to a very low-salt WFPBD diet and that problem has vanished. I've experienced other remarkable changes as well, such as little to no swelling or stiffness in my fingers, feet, or legs upon awakening. On the occasions that I go out to eat at restaurants where the food is salty, I clearly notice a difference as those problems return again. I've passed these tips onto many of my patients over the years and have received many happy responses, especially from people who have been able to get off their high blood pressure medications using these techniques.

SALT REPLACEMENTS	CONVERSION AMOUNTS
ORGANIC SOY and SOY DERIVATIVES like MISO, LOW SODIUM SOY SAUCE, or TAMARI can be used to replace or buffer table salt in cooking and are used in many soups, stews, Asian dishes, and pasta. **LIGHT MISO** is milder, less salty, and sweeter. **DARK MISO** is saltier and less sweet. Add miso toward the end of cooking as heat destroys the helpful fermented organisms it contains. Miso and soy have been shown to reduce and possibly prevent the hypertensive vessel damage and some cancer caused by salt.	Miso equivalents vary based on variety. 1 TBSP is equal to about 1/4-1/2 tsp salt. **MISO PASTE** is used for liquid and solid food recipes by adding a little warm water to make it pourable (a slurry). One bowl of miso soup equals about 1/4 tsp salt. **LOW SODIUM SOY SAUCE** works well in liquid recipes. **SOY POWDER** works well in combination with salt in dry recipes in roughly a one-to-one salt to soy ratio. Keep salt/sodium levels to a minimum. 1 tsp salt = 2,000-2,360 mg. 1 tsp of soy sauce = 180-300 m. 1 tsp miso = 200-300 mg sodium. Health agency regulated limit is 2,300 mg/day and even that is too high.
Fruits such as **LIME AND LEMON** make a good salt replacement or distraction for taste buds in many meals such as stews, soups, and chilis.	1 TBSP **LEMON JUICE** to replace 1/4 tsp salt - amount best determined by personal taste.
Vegetables such as **CELERY, GARLIC, CAPERS, YELLOW ONIONS, CHARD, AND SPINACH** provide a salty flavor.	All of these have various levels of saltiness and are best determined by personal taste. Start out with a small amount and increase as desired.
Consider adding **SEA VEGETABLES LIKE WAKAME, ALARIA, KOMBU, DULCE, KELP (small amount in powder form), SPIRULINA, NORI** to salads, soups, or stews, to add a salty seafood flavor and provide excellent nutrients such as omega oil and iodine.	**SEA VEGETABLES** vary in the amount of flavor, saltiness, and nutrients. Start out with a small amount and increase to the desired taste (limit amount of kelp powder to a pinch-very potent).
LEMONGRASS adds a nice salty flavor and is very popular in Asian dishes. Use the inner core by peeling away woodier outer layers. Cut into very thin rounds or slit stalk cores lengthwise and twist to release inner flavor and place in soups, other Asian dishes, or anything else you want.	1 TBSP minced **LEMONGRASS** may be equivalent to 1 TBSP lemon - best determined by recipe and personal taste.
HERBS AND SPICES such as **OREGANO, CILANTRO, CORIANDER SEED, PARSLEY, BLACK PEPPER, CAYENNE, DILL, CUMIN, AND PAPRIKA** all add saltiness. **BASIL** and **CARDAMON** are sweet & salty. These spices work well in Italian and Mexican dishes, pasta, pizza, stews, soups, and sauces to help replace the need for salt.	All of these have various levels of salty flavor and are best determined by the recipe and personal taste.
HOT SAUCES and **SALSA** are great for adding flavor to dishes to decrease the need for salt. Check salsa and hot sauce labels for sodium and chemical content and consider making your own. It is much simpler than you may think.	These have varying levels of saltiness and are best determined by health and personal taste.

SUBSTITUTING OIL AND BUTTER

Replace oil for sautéing or "frying" by using a little low sodium vegetable stock, broth, or water, or by omitting them altogether. Onions and many other vegetables actually have some natural oils in them. You will be surprised when you slowly sauté onions over medium heat to see that they caramelize beautifully without any added oil and you can eventually get used to cooking this way.

Vegetable stock and broth are excellent for adding richer flavor and more nutrients to your meals. They are usually made from parsley, bay leaves, carrots, celery, onion, cauliflower, broccoli, thyme, and pepper. Vegetable broth is generally lighter in color and often involves using trimmed vegetables, rice, and barley. It is boiled for about an hour and seasoned for drinking or as an instant soup. Vegetable stock typically involves sautéing vegetables, including their roots, skins, and stems. It is not usually seasoned and is often cooked commercially for up to forty-eight hours, making it thicker, darker, and richer. Save all your vegetable scraps, including pieces you cut off like washed roots, stems, etc., and keep them in a plastic bag in the freezer. Once you have enough, place them in a pot, add water, and boil for an hour or so to transform them into a homemade stew or soup. Remove the scraps once the nutrients are released, or even better, blend or purée some whole cooked vegetables in a large pot of water to make the ultimate healthy stock. See recipe for making your own vegetable stock at home.

It is best to wean yourself off of butter and butter substitutes and use hummus and avocado as spreads instead; but if you need to have something on a butter dish that your butter-loving family and friends will enjoy in place of butter, consider a cultured butter made primarily from oats or nuts or even vegan butter, which I hesitate to suggest which is made from a combination of extracted oil with the intention of balancing omega fatty oils. These can help some people with butter addictions improve their cholesterol levels, but they do not eliminate heart disease. Other substitutes for butter/fat are avocado and coconut cream, though coconut is higher in saturated fat.

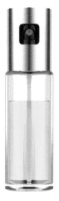

If you must use oil for cooking, only use a smidgen in the form of a spray or spritzer with a high smoke point like avocado oil and use extra virgin olive for non-heating purposes. Consider ordering a food-safe spray bottle for your oil instead of purchasing store-bought cooking sprays, which often contain chemical propellants and others unhealthy products. For baking, swapping out half of your oil with a vegetable like avocado is a step in the right direction. The other half of the oil can be replaced with a nut butter like cashew, walnut, peanut, or seed butter like tahini (sesame seeds). Consider unsweetened applesauce in nonsweet recipes and bananas in sweeter recipes where banana is a welcome flavor for replacing half of the oil. Baking fries or using an air fryer is a healthy way to make oil-free fries and other food typically cooked with oils. If desired, you can toss your fries in a miso slurry and dust with nutritional yeast for a healthier, buttery, cheesy, salty flavor.

Substituting with Nuts and Seeds

Nut butters from peanuts, walnuts, and cashews work well to replace butter/fat in cookies and other baked goods. Cashew butter has a sweet, subtle flavor and can be used to make cheese, creamy soups and sauces, coffee/tea creamers, and dessert creams.

For those with a strong genetic cholesterol disorder, this may mean an even more serious limit on their consumption, but keep in mind that flaxseeds and walnuts are well known to have some significant health benefits as well. Though nuts and seeds have many health benefits and are as tasty as they can be, keep consumption of them to a minimum. The general rule of thumb for plant food containing oil or fat is to limit portions of nuts, seeds, olives, avocados, and coconuts that contain even "healthy" monounsaturated or unsaturated fat. Extra fat of any type is stored in your body in places you won't want it.

Participants who consumed no more than three servings per week of walnuts had a 47 percent lower risk of cardiovascular mortality than those who did not consume walnuts. Also observed was that consuming walnuts at least once per week was associated with a 19 percent lower risk of cardiovascular disease, a 21 percent lower risk of coronary heart disease, and a 17 percent lower risk of stroke[59].

When buying nuts, keep in mind that blanching and roasting may damage the nutrients, so reach for raw, unblanched, natural nuts with no or low salt. When choosing nut butter, avoid those that have added refined oil, sugar, and salt. Make your own nut butter at home in your food processor or blender. Ideally, you can leave out added salt and sugar or add smaller amounts or healthier alternatives like miso paste or other soy in place of salt and more nutritive sweeteners like date syrup, molasses, honey, or pure maple syrup. Seed butter can be found in most stores, or as stated earlier, you can make your own by blending raw unroasted seeds. It takes about 10 minutes to turn seeds into a butter. Just get past the point where it is a paste in your blender by blending for about ten minutes.

Tahini (Sesame Seed Butter)

Tahini is butter or paste made from ground sesame seeds and can be added to recipes where you want to get some creaminess. It is rich in minerals, protein, calcium, vitamin E, B vitamins, fiber, iron, magnesium, and zinc. It may also improve healthy skin and cell growth. It is an excellent complement to miso paste, in many recipes, especially in sauces over noodles, soups, or dipping. It is commonly used in Middle Eastern dishes, such as hummus, falafel, or vinaigrettes, but it can also be put on fresh vegetables or fruit for a snack or bread as a delicious nutty-flavored non-nut spread. It works well as a butter replacement for making garlic bread as well. Make your own tahini at home with hulled white sesame seeds. Just place them in a food processor and blend for about ten minutes, scraping sides along the way. No other ingredients are needed—just a little patience.

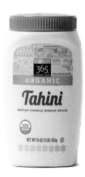

Vegetable and Fruit Purées in Place of Oil

You can have so much fun creating low-fat, healthy sauces, and dressings by replacing oil with puréed fruit and vegetables. Fruit is delicious mixed with some balsamic or lemon juice, herbs, and water. Fruit and veggie purées can make meal presentation very impressive by adding drizzles of color. Consider using silken tofu, a neutral flavor, cauliflower, nuts, or seeds to adjust flavor and color, and add creaminess.

Healthy Replacement Options:

Carrot or pumpkin purée: is a beautiful orange color you can use as a sauce on whole rice or pasta. Sprinkle some fresh parsley or other favorite herb or spice for a gourmet accent.

Corn purée: provides a sweet flavor and yellow tint and is especially suitable for thickening vinaigrettes.

Pea purée: is another idea for incorporating healthy legumes in sauces. Don't overcook them. Add fresh green herbs like parsley, kale, spinach, or mint to make for a brighter or darker green color while adding more flavor with herbs and spices and added nutrients.

Red bell pepper purée: provides sweetness and red coloring. Roasting red bell peppers first gives them a smoky flavor.

Red beets: for that lovely, deep purple-red color can be combined with anything, including tofu or corn, to make beautiful dressings and sauces.

Blueberries: for that deep purple antioxidant blue, make for a terrific sauce on pancakes or desserts. They are also delicious, combined with herbs and spices and vinegar for a salad dressing.

Apple purée: makes an excellent flavor for vinaigrette dressings and sweet sauces.

Mangos, raspberries, and strawberries: are also great in vinaigrettes and as sauces for desserts.

Cocoa powder, 100%: mixed with maple syrup, avocado, or tofu makes a creamy, delicious sauce for everything.

OIL REPLACEMENTS	CONVERSION AMOUNTS
VEGETABLE STOCK, BROTH, or **WATER** plus **NUTRITIONAL YEAST, VINEGAR, LEMON** or **LIME JUICE** and a small amount of **XANTHAN GUM** can be used to thicken and stabilize liquids for salad dressings.	**XANTHAN GUM POWDER** - 1/4 tsp per cup of liquid + 1 ½ teaspoons nutritional yeast to make an oil-like liquid. No need to cook xanthan, but 5-10 minutes wait time is required for thickening.
CHIA SEEDS or FLAXSEEDS can be used to thicken many foods such as puddings, sauces, and gravies. Flaxseeds release their nutritional content when blended, crushed, or chewed. Chia seed pudding is a very popular healthy dessert and resembles tapioca pudding in texture but is far superior in nutrition.	**CHIA SEEDS** For an oil-like consistency, 1 TBSP per 1 cup liquid, allow to set for 10 minutes. For egg-like gel consistency use 1 TBSP chia seeds + 3 TBSP water. For pudding, 1 part chia seeds to 4 parts liquid. Allow two hours for whole seeds to fully absorb liquid.
NUT and SEED BUTTERS - Peanut butter, sesame seed butter (tahini), cashew butter/cream, walnut butter, pumpkin seed butter, pecan butter, add creaminess to salad dressings and sauces.	**NUT** or **SEED BUTTER** + water + vinegar or citrus juice for salad dressings. Increase liquid by 2-3 times to compensate for increased fiber content.
AVOCADO or **PUMPKIN PURÉE** can be used in place of oil, butter, and eggs in baking and adds natural creaminess to anything when green color is acceptable. Avocado complements food containing cocoa/chocolate very nicely.	Replace 1 cup oil with 1 cup **PUMPKIN or AVOCADO PURÉE** and increase liquid or decrease dry ingredients by 15-20% to compensate for increased fiber content.
ONION can be pureed fresh or caramelized and pureed to add thickening and flavoring to salad dressings, gravies, sauces, soups, or stews.	3 TBSP fresh (blended) or 1/2 cup caramelized onion per 1 cup liquid (salad dressing, gravy, sauce, soup, or stew).
CAULIFLOWER can be used to make creamy sauces for pastas, mixed with some nut or seed butter and water.	Replace oil with equal amount of cooked and blended cauliflower.
CORN PURÉE (cooked) can replace oil, provides a sweet flavor, a yellow tint, and is especially suitable for thickening vinaigrettes and gravies.	Replace oil with an equal amount of corn puree.
SILKEN TOFU for salad dressing or sauces to thicken or add creaminess.	Use in place of oil (and water) in creamy salad dressings.
WHITE BEANS or **POTATOES** (cooked) can be used for salad dressing or sauces to thicken and add creaminess.	Replace oil with cooked and puréed beans or potatoes, adding water to desired consistency.
BANANAS provide plenty of nutrients, decrease calorie and fat content, and can substitute eggs, oil, butter, and sugar when a banana flavor is acceptable.	Add an equal amount of pureed banana to replace oil or butter (replace only one recipe ingredient).
APPLE SAUCE and **SWEET POTATO PURÉE** can be used as a replacement for eggs, oil, butter, and sugar, depending on the recipe.	Replace oil or butter with an equal amount of unsweetened apple sauce. Consider reducing other sweeteners in recipe.
DATE PASTE can substitute oil or butter instead of banana to avoid a banana flavor (add sweetness to cookies, muffins, and other baked goods).	Replace oil or butter with an equal amount of puréed dates (heated, soaked/softened). Consider reducing other sweeteners in the recipe.
AGAR POWDER (or flakes) is made from seaweed, is colorless and odorless, and must be simmered in liquid for 5 minutes to activate thickening/gelling properties. It is often used in place of gelatin to thicken gravies, soups, preserves, puddings, custards, meringue, and jello.	For thickening gravy, use 1 teaspoon agar per 1 cup of liquid. For a jello consistency, use 1 1/2 tablespoons per cup of liquid. For heating nondairy milk to an egg white consistency use 2 teaspoons per cup.

BUTTER REPLACEMENTS	CONVERSION AMOUNTS
APPLE SAUCE (unsweetened) contains 100 calories per cup, while butter contains about 1600 calories per cup. Apple sauce can be used to replace butter in baked goods like muffins, cookies, cakes, bread, pancakes, and brownies.	Replace half of the butter with apple sauce and the other half with tofu or non-dairy yogurt to reduce sweetness and increase nutrient variety or reduce the amount of the other sweeteners in the recipe. Add a pinch of salt, miso slurry, or soy sauce to replace salted butter taste (optional).
NUT or SEED BUTTERS - Peanut butter, sesame seed butter (tahini), cashew butter, walnut butter, pumpkin seed butter, and pecan butter can be used in place of butter in baked goods.	Replace butter with an equal amount of nut or seed butter of similar consistency. Add a pinch of salt, miso slurry, or soy sauce to replace salted butter taste (optional). May need to reduce amount of flour/dry ingredients by 10-15%.
PUMPKIN PURÉE and SWEET POTATO PURÉE can be used as a replacement for butter, and some sugar, depending on the recipe.	Replace 1 cup butter with 3/4 cup or 20-25% less pumpkin or sweet potato puree. Add a pinch of salt, miso, or soy sauce to replace salted butter taste, optional. Consider reducing other sweet ingredients in the recipe.
NUTRITIONAL YEAST or "Nooch" is a product used for making nondairy cheese, has a mild nuttiness, and is also used to replace butter. Can be used as a regular source of B12. Check the label to verify content.	Use nutritional yeast to sprinkle on pasta, popcorn, or on anything welcoming a buttery, cheesy, slightly nutty flavor. For making nondairy "Parmesan cheese," combine 1 cup blended cashews or hemp seeds, 1/4 cup nutritional yeast, 3/4 tsp salt, 1/4 tsp garlic powder, and 3/4 tsp soy powder to help buffer salt.
BANANAS can be used to substitute butter and sugar when a banana flavor is acceptable. They provide plenty of nutrients and significantly decrease fat content.	Use an equal amount of banana to replace butter or use 1/2 silken tofu and 1/2 banana. Consider reducing other sweeteners to compensate for sweetness of banana.
DATE PASTE can be used to replace butter and sugar when wanting to avoid a banana flavor. It adds sweetness to any baked goods including cookies, muffins, and brownies.	Date paste is made by blending an equal number of pitted dates with warm water. Consider reducing other sweeteners in the recipe.
AVOCADO adds creaminess and complements chocolate in food like chocolate smoothies and brownies. Use it in recipes with a darker color or when a green color is acceptable.	Use an equal amount of pureed avocado to replace the butter. Add a pinch of salt, miso slurry, or soy sauce to replace salted butter taste, optional.
HUMMUS can be used to substitute butter and mayonnaise on sandwiches and wraps.	Use an equal amount and add a pinch of salt, miso slurry, or soy sauce to replace salted butter taste, optional.
With great hesitation, I list **EARTH BALANCE and SMART BALANCE** as examples of butter substitutes. They are made with a combination of oil said to be from plants. To make oil a butter-like solid, it is usually hydrogenated creating trans fats. It may be a lower-fat product than butter and can help some people who are hooked on butter improve their cholesterol levels, but it does not eliminate heart disease. These are not whole food. They contain other chemicals and they are man-made - need I say more? If you use it, use limited amounts and consider using hummus, avocado, or a nut butter as a spread for your bread instead.	In baking or cooking, use a little less "plant-based" buttery spread to replace butter as it melts more thinly. Most of these spreads do not handle higher heat well, so add them last. Earth balance comes in the form of a butter stick shape which may be a good product to keep on a butter dish for guests and for thinly spreading on bread and pancakes, to taste/health.

SUBSTITUTING SUGAR

The most common form of sugar in America is white table sugar. It is highly refined, high in unhealthy calories offering no nutritional benefit, has a very high glycemic index, and studies show that consuming it can, in fact, shorten your life.

Brown sugar is no better than white sugar when it comes to nutritional quality. Brown sugar is simply white table sugar very lightly coated with some molasses to add a darker color and more flavor.

Highly refined sweeteners are well known to be involved in worsening or causing inflammatory diseases, especially, diabetes.

Many quick commercial food sources like granola bars and yogurt contain about 12 grams of added sugar per serving and most sugary drinks have at least 40 grams sugar per serving. It is best to avoid processed or refined sugar when possible.

Whole food sources like fruit, including date sugar, date paste, bananas, unsweetened applesauce, pumpkin puree, dried fruit like raisins, apricots, cherries, maple, molasses, and honey are all healthier alternatives for sugar. Other healthy options that can trick your mind as sweetening options are natural vanilla, cinnamon, ginger, cloves, basil, or nutmeg. They enhance flavor, give the illusion of sweetness, and they all have unique health benefits. Combine these with healthy grains like oats and nuts or seeds to make your own healthy treats.

Some people find it difficult to eliminate refined sweeteners, but once taste buds are retrained or adjusted to natural 'whole' sweeteners, most people find that they enjoy, and even crave them equally as much. Whole sweetening sources contain natural nutritional content, including fiber which slows sugar/carb absorption reducing the glycemic index, making it an excellent alternative, especially for diabetics.

Sugar Cane: Turbinado, Demerara, Muscovado (and Beet Sugar)

The sugar cane plant in its raw natural form contains nutrient-rich molasses syrup which is removed from the plant during processing. To be sold as what is called "raw sugar " or " organic cane sugar," the sugar cane plant goes through an extensive refining process that depletes it of most of its nutrients. Turbinado, Muscovado, and Demerara are also refined. To convert these sugars into a more to a crystallized form, they are refined even more. Like "organic cane sugar," "organic beet sugar" is also refined and when crystallized from the original plant, it has little to no nutritional value. The rule of thumb is, the darker the color, the more molasses and nutrients they typically contain.

Bananas

In baking, bananas can be used as a substitute for oil, eggs, and sugar, where a sweet banana flavor is acceptable. As mentioned earlier, they are high in fiber, potassium, calcium, and prebiotics. They can help with acid reflux, high blood pressure, balancing electrolytes, and even mood stabilization. They are a great replacement in cookies, muffins, cakes, and bread. Replace 1/2 of the oil in baked goods with an equal amount of mashed banana and replace the other half with tofu, nondairy yogurt, or other less sweet option (See Oil Replacements chart.)

Applesauce

Applesauce is another suitable baking replacement for oil in cookies, muffins, cakes, bread, and brownies. It has about 100 calories per cup, while vegetable oils have approximately 2,080 calories per cup. Use an unsweetened apple sauce as a substitute for butter, eggs, and oil for making muffins, cookies, cakes, bread, and brownies. It is also great in pancakes and as a topping with cinnamon, raisins, nuts, and seeds for oatmeal. It has a relatively long shelf life, offers a lot of fiber, vitamin C, and is very low in fat and calories. Apples contain antioxidants that prevent cell damage and lower asthma risk, Alzheimer's, cancer, and heart disease. They can also help control type 1 diabetes and reduce the risk for type 2 diabetes and many other inflammatory disorders. You can make applesauce yourself easily at home in a slow cooker or on the stovetop.

Medjool Dates, Date Paste, and Date Syrup (Nature's Caramel)

Medjool dates are possibly the sweetest, tastiest, most nutritious, and most versatile of all dried fruit. They come in the form of a sugar, a paste, or a syrup which is often referred to as nature's natural caramel. Dates are a delicious addition to your oatmeal, granola, smoothie, or dessert and offer an abundance of vitamins, minerals, protein, antioxidants, and fiber. The high fiber content provides a low glycemic index resulting in a sustained energy release without the sugar crash. Dates regulate bowel movements, help fight colon cancer, and possibly help prevent prostate, lung, and breast cancer. They can be used in baked goods in place of sugar, brown sugar, oil, and butter. In their purest form, dates are very rich in fiber, and as a paste they have a thick, fibrous consistency. Date paste syrup is considered the most nutritious of all syrup sweeteners, and molasses comes in as a close second. Some of the fiber can be removed, making it more like a syrup that is often used in place of molasses, maple syrup, caramel, and honey. Date syrup containing its fiber does not dissolve well in coffee or tea. Make date paste by blending pitted dates with some water.

Maple Syrup

Pure maple syrup is well-known as a natural sugar substitute and is a healthier alternative to table sugar. It is heated at high temperatures to make it thicker but retains some nutrients. It contains minerals such as calcium, iron, magnesium, zinc, some B vitamins, antioxidants, and also contains prebiotic oligosaccharides that help to feed the good flora or bacteria in your digestive system. Maple sugar is sweeter than regular sugar, so in baking, you can use about 2/3 cup maple sugar for every cup of regular sugar and reduce liquid by about 20 percent or by 2 tablespoons for every half cup of maple syrup added. Pure maple syrup is versatile and can be used in combination with dates in sauces, pancakes, hot chocolate, salad dressings, and oatmeal. You can also use it to glaze vegetables, fruit, and desserts.

Agave Nectar

Agave nectar is marketed as a safe alternative to sugar for people with diabetes, but the nutritional value of agave is nearly zero. Agave nectar is obtained from the agave plant and processed using high heat to separate it from its fiber content and most of its nutrients. It has the same nonnutritional value as white table sugar, corn syrup, and brown rice syrup.

Honey

Pure raw honey is usually not put through the same high heat and separation process as agave and contains some phytonutrients including vitamin C, vitamin E, minerals, antioxidants, and prebiotic oligosaccharides. Honey is known for its antibacterial effects, accelerating wound healing, treating mouth ulcers, and having some antidiabetic effects. Many store-bought honey products are pasteurized to kill bacteria and are mixed with high fructose corn syrup, so check labels and select honey in its purest form. Your local farmers are likely going to be the best source.

Avoid Processed Sweeteners and Sugars

Many store-bought, processed sweeteners such as Equal, Splenda, Sweet'N Low, NutraSweet, and Benevia contain, or are made from, high-fructose corn syrup, fructose syrup, dextrose, malt, maltodextrin, saccharin, sucralose, aspartame, acesulfame-K, and evaporated cane juice, which is just as void of nutrients as white sugar. These sweeteners have varying degrees of detrimental effects such as the development of cancer and tumor growth, thyroid damage resulting in weight gain, nausea, headaches, mood swings, heart palpitations, hypoglycemia, liver and kidney impairment, Alzheimer's, Parkinson's, vision damage, insomnia, diarrhea, joint pain, multiple sclerosis, premature births, and babies with brain cancer. It is best to avoid all artificial sweeteners. They increase your cravings and addictions to super-sweet tasting food. Fortunately, it takes only three weeks of abstinence from artificial sweeteners to eliminate cravings and psychological dependence on them.

In summary, the healthiest sweeteners are fruit-mainly dates (date paste or date sugar, containing both soluble and insoluble fiber), pineapple, apples, grapes, blueberries, and pomegranate, just to name a few. Date sugar, date paste, and molasses are the healthiest concentrated sweeteners, with dates being more nutritious than molasses, which is partially processed by separating it from the cane plant. Pure honey and pure maple syrup are the next healthiest 'syrup' sweeteners, though they are a drop in nutrition compared to dates and molasses.

Stevia

Stevia is extracted from the stevia leaves of the stevia plant, but when sold commercially, it usually contains highly refined chemicals such as erythritol, dextrose, and maltodextrin. Many of these have been proven unsafe, so it is likely best to avoid these items. Because stevia is said to be fifty times sweeter than sugar, has no calories, and no glycemic index, the commercial brands are widely used especially among diabetics throughout Europe, Japan, South and North America. These extracted and processed forms are not considered "whole food," but you can actually grow your own stevia plants in their "whole food" form at home. You simply mash the leaves in the bottom of your cup to sweeten tea and coffee. The leaves are very sweet and delicious!

SUGAR REPLACEMENTS	CONVERSION AMOUNTS
DATE SUGAR contains quite a bit of fiber and can be used in place of brown sugar or white sugar in baked goods such as cookies, bread, muffins, and brownies or in any dish some fiber can hide in. Honey and maple syrup work better in liquids such as tea or coffee.	Use date sugar in place of white or brown sugar in a one-to-one ratio.
DATE PASTE can be used to replace sugar in baked goods like cookies and muffins. Add equal amounts of pitted dates and hot water to a blender and blend to a creamy paste.	Use about 3/4 cup date paste for every cup of granulated sugar and reduce recipe liquid (milk or water) by about 10% or about 1 1/2 TBSP for every cup.
DATE SYRUP/DATE CARAMEL is used as a topping on oatmeal, cereal, ice cream, and in smoothies. It is darker in color when heated and fiber is partially removed. Date syrup is considered the most nutritious of all syrup sweeteners and molasses comes in as a close second.	Use equal amounts in place of molasses, maple syrup, or honey. Make date syrup by adding 1-part pitted dates to 1 1/2 parts water. Adjust to desired consistency. Removing the fiber is not recommended.
PURE MAPLE SYRUP is heated at high temperatures but retains some nutrients. It is used in sauces, salad dressings, desserts, hot chocolate, pancakes, oatmeal, and for glazing vegetables and fruit.	In baking, use 2/3 cup maple syrup, date syrup, or honey for every cup of sugar and reduce recipe liquid (milk or water) by 20-25%.
PURE HONEY contains antioxidants and other nutrients that support your microbiome. It is a good sweetener for whiter or lighter colored foods such as "mayonnaise" or light-colored sauces and frostings.	In baking, use 2/3 cup honey, date syrup, or maple syrup for every cup of sugar. Increase dry ingredients by 20% or reduce recipe liquid (milk or water) by 20%.
APPLE SAUCE can be used to replace sugar in baking and for making sauces and dressings.	When using apple sauce to replace sugar, reduce the amount of other liquid (milk or water) in the recipe by 20%.
BANANAS can be used to substitute sugar when baking cookies, muffins, cakes, bread, brownies, and blending smoothies or ice cream when a banana flavor is acceptable.	Use puréed bananas to reduce sugar by reducing the amount of liquid in the recipe by 20%. Consider reducing sweeteners in the recipe to compensate for banana sweetness.
FRUIT PUREES, including dates, pumpkin, raisin, and apples can replace sugar in baked goods, desserts, sauces, and syrups.	Use about 3/4 cup purée for every cup of granulated sugar and reduce recipe liquid (milk or water) by about 10% or about 1 1/2 TBSP for every cup.
ONIONS - Fresh sweet onions, purple onions, and shallots can be used to thicken salad dressings. Cooked or caramelized onions can be used to thicken gravy and sauces.	Use 2-3 TBSP of fresh chopped onion to blend into 1 cup of salad dressing liquid. For gravy and sauces, add 1 cup cooked onion to 1 cup liquid.
HERBS AND SPICES that provide some degree of sweetness include basil, stevia leaves, cinnamon, cloves, mint, cilantro/coriander, paprika, dill, fennel, cardamom, nutmeg, mace, ginger, vanilla, parsley, chives, and tarragon.	Herbs and spices vary in amounts depending on combination of ingredients in your recipe and your taste.
RAW ORGANIC CANE SUGAR (Demerara, Muscovado and **Turbinado)** and **RAW ORGANIC BEET SUGAR** can be used to replace table sugar, though not considered nutritious. To cut down on the amount used, consider using dates, bananas, or applesauce in baked goods and sprinkle or lightly coat baked goods with cane sugar crystals.	Equal amounts, depending on granule size. Large crystals may require some semi-grinding or crushing for some recipes.
STEVIA plants can be home grown, and the leaves can be used in a "whole food" form. Leaves can be crushed or blended to sweeten teas and coffees.	Stevia is said to be fifty times sweeter than sugar. Adjust to taste.

Fruit Juice Concentrates and Pure Fruit Juice

Many doctors advise against drinking commercial fruit juice because of the high glycemic index, processed sugar content, and the lack of nutrients. One of the most dangerous forms of sweeteners, high fructose corn syrup, is often added to fruit juice, especially frozen jucie concentrate. High fructose corn syrup is strongly linked to metabolic complications like type 2 diabetes, cardiac disease, belly fat accumulation, and high triglyceride levels. Those who choose store bought juice should be sure to select one hundred percent "pure" fruit juice but realize that even most of the best brands have at least some fiber and nutrients removed or damaged through processing.

On the other hand, fruit juiced from its original "whole" form (oranges, lemons, grapefruit, apples, etc.), preserving the pith and pulp, contain nutrients and insoluble fiber. You can make your own fruit juice by removing the thicker (tough) skin and blending them into a purée, adding some water, as needed. Sweeten sour fruit with grapes, pineapple, apples, berries, or other natural sweeteners. Many people find it difficult to drink plain water, and fruit intake is one of the most neglected nutrient sources in our diets. But an easy way to increase water and fruit intake is by combining them. I've been "watering down" my juice for nearly 30 years with water since learning this trick while pregnant with my first child. My obstetrician advised that I do that as my weight was getting out of control, early on. Genetics! Ugh! You too can do this, and your taste will adjust. Before you know it, the sweet flavor of store-bought juices will become repulsive.

CHEESE SUBSTITUTES

Alternatives such as cauliflower, tofu, potatoes, and white beans are excellent options for making cheese, cheese sauces, gravies, and desserts. Cashews can be blended to a cream as well and has a deliciously creamy flavor and texture, but the fat content can be quite high if portions are not limited.

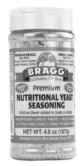

Nutritional Yeast, AKA "Nooch"

Nutritional yeast is a complete protein containing about 2 grams of protein in 1 tablespoon. It has a hint of hearty nuttiness and typically contains an abundance of B12 and many other vitamins and minerals. Many varieties of nutritional yeast have more than 575 percent of the RDA of vitamin B12. It is a delicious staple in plant-based and vegan diets, adding excellent cheesy flavor and many health benefits. Most people don't have a problem eating any amount of nutritional yeast, but for some eating more than a tablespoon may trigger a headache. Nutritional yeast can increase energy, support your immune system, reduce inflammation, improve skin conditions, reduce cold symptoms, and may lower blood glucose levels and cholesterol.

According to some of Dr. Greger's review studies, nutritional yeast is often recommended to athletes for boosting their immune system[60]. It has also been shown help reduce breast cancer and promote wound healing[61]. New studies show that 1/16th of a teaspoon (a pinch) of nutritional yeast can cut common childhood respiratory illnesses by 40 percent and reduce illness time to three days.

Add nutritional yeast to your salt-seasoning replacement shaker to have on hand for use on anything. It is the key ingredient for flavoring homemade plant-based cheese. It is combined with ground cashews or hemp seeds, garlic, and salt to make a "parmesan cheese" replacement that can be shaken liberally on food such as spaghetti, pizza, popcorn, roasted vegetables, salads, and kale chips. Nutritional yeast is also used to make creamy cheese sauces for pasta, rice dishes, casseroles, mashed potatoes, and so much more. Ingredients vary between brands, so check labels to make sure it meets nutritional needs. People with Crohn's disease and gluten sensitivities should use caution with nutritional yeast as they may experience an immune response due to their avoidance of bread containing yeast. More reliable purity brands containing B12 are Bob's Red Mill, Bragg, Red Star, and Dr. Fuhrman's, but again, check the labels to be sure.

EGG SUBSTITUTES

You can make plant-based scrambled "eggs" with tofu, egg flavoring, and turmeric, an incredible cancer fighter that adds a bright yellow color. Kala Namak is a light pink colored, sulfurized salt that smells and tastes like egg. Though salt is considered unhealthy, a small amount applied to tofu "eggs" is rather insignificant compared to how much salt (and other health-damaging products) you are eliminating from your diet by no longer eating processed food, meat, eggs, or dairy products. Additionally, many studies seem to show that soy counters the damaging effects to vessels from salt/sodium intake by reducing hypertension and other related complications.

Some of the best plant-based "scrambled eggs" can be made from pre-frozen silken tofu or unfrozen firm tofu. Tofu is usually soaked in and packaged in water. Soft or silken tofu has a curd like texture, but freezing it makes it easier to press when removing the water and it also causes some shrinking and a firmer texture, making it very much like that of scrambled eggs. Unfrozen, firm, pressed tofu can crumble into an egg-like texture as well but is more firm than typical scrambled eggs. Both ways will amaze you! After pressing, heat up a skillet over medium heat, crumble the tofu over it, sprinkle tofu with turmeric and Kala Namak, toss to coat, and heat through. Unlike dairy eggs, which can often carry salmonella, organic tofu from reliable suppliers is precooked and can actually be eaten raw. I'll share more information about tofu later in this chapter.

Egg replacement products intended for baking are available in stores that are quite popular but are typically composed of processed ingredients. Some are made from whole legumes like chickpeas, but the healthiest option for replacing eggs in baking are flaxseed, chia seed, and many others (see Egg Replacements chart). Chia seeds and flaxseeds need to be ground, crushed, or chewed to release their nutrient supply. When added to liquids and allowed to set, they become a or egg-like substance.

EGG REPLACEMENTS	CONVERSION AMOUNTS
CRUSHED FLAXSEED or CHIA SEEDS are an excellent replacement for eggs in baked goods such as cookies, brownies, muffins, or cakes. They provide protein, fiber, omega oil, anti-cancer lignans, improve brain function, decrease heart disease risk, help reverse or decrease diabetes and many other inflammatory and immune diseases.	1 TBSP crushed flaxseed or chia seeds + 3 TBSP water, let set for 5-10 minutes to gel for replacing one egg.
APPLE SAUCE can replace eggs or oil when baking but may not work well to replace both in the same recipe.	1/4 cup apple sauce to replace one egg.
BANANAS can be used to substitute eggs, oil, and/or sugar when a banana flavor is acceptable but may not work well to replace all three in the same recipe.	1/2 mashed or 1/4 cup pureed banana to replace one egg.
PURÉED FRUIT can be used in any baked goods to replace egg and to add flavor and nutrients.	Use 1/4 cup pureed fruit for replacing one egg.
OATS can be blended to a powder and cooked to a gooey consistency for use in any baked goods. You can also cook oats first then blend to a creamy custard.	Use 1/4 cup cooked and blended (or unblended) oats to replace one egg.
TOFU can be used in any baked goods, custards, or creamy shakes.	1/4 cup silken tofu, unfrozen with some water removed to replace one egg.
Previously frozen **SILKEN TOFU** is an excellent replacement for scrambled eggs.	See recipe.
MASHED POTATO AND SWEET POTATO can be used in baked goods or sauces for egg replacement.	1/4 cup mashed potato or sweet potato to replace one egg. Consider reducing other sweet ingredients.
CAULIFLOWER, cooked and blended to a cream can be use in baked goods or sauces to replace eggs.	1/4 cup cauliflower to replace one egg.
NON-DAIRY PLAIN YOGURT can be used in baked goods, desserts, custards, or smoothies for replacing egg.	Use 1/4 cup plain, non-dairy yogurt to replace one egg.
TOMATO PASTE is a suitable egg replacement in food like "meatloaves" and burgers where color is not important.	Use 3-4 TBSP of tomato paste to replace one egg.

Milk Substitutes

The variety of nondairy milk and creamers now available at our local grocery stores is amazing, but I initially found it hard to convince my son to switch from dairy milk to nondairy milk, especially since dairy milk is the only choice offered at our public schools. It took some time to help him understand the health benefits and differences between them, but after quite extensively exploring the varieties available, he eventually found some that work for him. We tried everything, including combinations of various flavors in an attempt to neutralize any particular taste. The varieties include sweetened and unsweetened almond milk, coconut milk, soy milk, banana milk, pea milk and more. My son's favorite is vanilla almond milk with a touch of honey (honey should be avoided with children under one year of age). Homemade almond milk is a great way to ensure your child's milk contains only the healthiest ingredients. Our family's overall nondairy milk choice started out as the dark chocolate almond milk. Try that one out with your chocolate-loving kids and friends! They will likely become hooked.

When the COVID-19 pandemic first broke, plenty of nondairy milk options were available in the stores, and people were complaining that the stores were running out of dairy milk. That made it very easy for us to find our favorite milk, but this lasted only for about a month as people began to learn about the health risks of inflammatory diseases or comorbidities associated with the virus. As their knowledge grew about the benefits of plant-based food, we noticed that the nondairy milk began to fly off the shelves, and suddenly there was plenty of dairy milk left behind. That's when we learned how to make homemade plant milk much lower in sweetener and salt, and with no additives.

When it comes to protein in nondairy milk, a wide gap exists between soy milk and other types of milk. Soy usually offers about 7 grams versus 1 to 3 grams of protein from others made from nuts, oats, and vegetables, but if you are consuming a WFPBD including legumes and grains, you should easily meet your protein needs either way.

Creamer Substitutes

Oat Creamer Powder for On the Go

Oat milk creamer found at some favorite coffee shops can be steamed up for a delicious, creamy, healthier dairy alternative. You can make your own at home by blending rolled oats into a fine powder using a coffee bean grinder or high power blender and adding water. Unfiltered oatmilk may leave sediment in the bottom of the cup. Sediment can be removed with a filter cloth and added back into your diet in smoothies or muffins. Place some oat powder in a baggie to take with you on the run to add to your coffee or tea.

Soy and Oat Creamer - Healthy and Delicious

A combination of silken soy and oats is another healthier nondairy creamer you can use in your coffee or tea. Place 1/2 block of soft or silken soy, 1/4 cup rolled oats, and 1/2 cup water in a high-powered blender and blend until creamy. Add pure maple syrup or another pure sweetener and store in the refrigerator for about a week.

Lowfat Coconut Milk/Cream - Delicious, but High in Fat

The American Heart Association (AHA) recommends consuming no more than 11 to 13 total grams of fat per day and does not recommend the use of coconut cream because it is high in saturated fat[62, 63]. Even in isolated populations where only whole coconuts are eaten in a plant-based diet, total cholesterol levels were over 200. To reduce the amount of fat when using coconut milk cream, use light or low fat, and consider cutting it in half with soy milk, oat milk.

MEAT SUBSTITUTES

Legumes (beans, peas, and lentils) and whole grains are a excellent options for replacing meat protein and adding plentiful nutrients to any meal. Soybeans have been shown to help reduce the damaging effects of salt on our vessels, which means it can help control or prevent hypertension. Soybeans also have many anticancer benefits. Tofu and tempeh are made from soybeans and absorb flavor very well. People are amazed with the meaty flavors that can be created from plant sources that can be added to sauces, lasagnas, chilies, and burgers. There are delectable replacement flavors for bacon, sausage, pepperoni, and seafood that will also amaze your family and friends. See section on *Complete Proteins* for other excellent high protein options.

Tofu

As stated earlier, tofu (soy) had a bad reputation for many years. The estrogen in soy is a *phyto*estrogen that actually competes with animal-sourced estrogen at receptors. It has been proven to prevent cancer in the human body versus the opposite as shown in other species originally tested. Even though tofu is partially processed, the soy curd is still packed with plenty of nutrients, including protein and iron. Tofu is very versatile and easily soaks up marinade and sauce flavors and is delicious when it is properly prepared. Organically prepared silken tofu from a reliable source can be used to make food like mayonnaise, creams, puddings, and sour cream. The easiest way to handle softer or silken tofu for cooking is to freeze it for about eight hours and no more than two weeks. The freeze/thaw method changes silken tofu to a more scrambled egg consistency and firm tofu texture becomes a firmer consistency like that of chicken. Tofu is packaged in water, and when frozen and thawed, it is very easy to squeeze the water out by hand. Unfrozen firm tofu can be pressed between weighted pots or plates to yield a less fibrous state that is very popular for baking/searing softer pieces and tofu crumbles. Keep tofu on hand to chop into small pieces to add protein to any stir-fry, soup, stew, casserole, quiche, curry, or pasta. Tofu can be baked, air fried, grilled, steamed, or pan-fried. You can also simply add soybeans or any other legume instead.

Soft or Silken Tofu

Silken tofu has the most water in it and has a very mild flavor with a custard-like texture. Use silken tofu for blending into smoothies, sauces, creams, and for making plant-based mayonnaise, sour cream, silken dips, creamy dressings, and desserts such as puddings. Removing the water from silken tofu is much more challenging than removing it from firmer forms of tofu, but it can be done with a terry cloth or dish towel. Pre-frozen, thawed, and gently squeezed, silken tofu is ideal for making scrambled eggs.

Firm or Extra Firm Tofu

Firm tofu is an excellent in stir-fries, curries, soups, and stews. Unfrozen firm tofu has a dense consistency that works well combined with plant-based cheese flavors blended in an artichoke dip or a broccoli cheddar dip. It is not as smooth and creamy as silken tofu.

As mentioned above, freezing and thawing tofu allows you to easily remove water by hand. Pressing tofu between plates or a saucepan weighted with water for 20 to 30 minutes. A tofu press is another tool used to remove water.

Frying or Searing and Tofu

There have long been concerns about Teflon-type non-stick cookware. Studies show that this type of cookware, when intact (not worn) and used with temperatures kept within the medium heat range does not release chemical toxins. If the cookware begins to chip or wear, the recommendation is to dispose of them. One hundred percent ceramic, stainless steel, or iron is considered the safest cookware to use.

Tempeh

Tempeh is a fermented, cooked soybean patty or loaf that may be combined with whole grains and is rich in probiotics, the beneficial microbes found in our digestive tracts. It is a complete protein and is significantly nutrient-dense. It has a grainier beanlike texture compared to tofu and a mildly nutty, earthy flavor. Like tofu, tempeh absorbs flavors and marinades but takes longer because it is denser. Tempeh must be soaked in marinade for at least an hour, overnight, or cooked in your sauces or stews for a deeper flavor. Try adding tempeh to a stir-fry instead of tofu if you have it on hand. It is an excellent replacement for ground beef as you can crumble it, chop it, add it to soup, spaghetti sauce, chili, lasagna, etc. Tempeh can be sliced and marinated in beef or chicken flavored bouillon and sautéed as part of a quick high protein meal. You can make tempeh taste very much like bacon with various seasonings including soy sauce, garlic, maple syrup, nutritional yeast, liquid smoke, and miso. See recipe section.

OTHER MEAT SUBSTITUTES

Jackfruit, Hearts of Palm, Mushrooms, Nuts and Seeds

Jackfruit is full of great health benefits. It is especially rich in vitamin C and fiber. The nutrients found in jackfruit help enhance immunity, support digestion, and improve heart health. It can be found fresh or canned and has a texture similar to chicken or pork. It is an excellent addition to plant-based meals. Most people prefer to buy it canned because working with fresh jackfruit is quite a sticky process and it can weigh up to a hundred pounds. Hearts of Palm is similar to jackfruit but has a nice white flaky texture making it a great stand in for fish and crab meat substitutes for food like ceviche and crabcakes.

Mushrooms are also an excellent way to add nutrients to any diet, and they are low in calories and have antioxidant and antimicrobial properties. Portobello, shiitake, and porcini mushrooms, in particular, add hearty, savory depth of flavor to any dish. Their meaty flavor works well for making burgers, stews, casseroles, and pasta dishes.

Nuts and seeds are high in healthy fat, fiber, vitamins, and minerals, so it should come as no surprise that they can help "beef" up your meals with many nutrients found in meat, eggs, and dairy. As stated earlier, studies show that a higher intake of nuts was associated with a lower risk of heart disease. Walnuts, almonds, Brazil nuts, cashews, flaxseeds, chia seeds, and hemp seeds are some of the healthiest nuts and seeds.

Seitan and Vital Wheat Gluten

Seitan has been a popular meat substitute among vegetarians and vegans for many years. It is considered the "white meat" of these diets and is often used in products sold as "plant-based" or "vegan." It consists of the main protein found in wheat—gluten. It is separated from the fiber and other nutrients and is sold as *vital wheat gluten*. Seitan or vital wheat gluten goes through an extensive refining process, and as mentioned earlier is not considered a whole food, nor is it considered healthy. Unlike tofu and tempeh, it does not typically contain any soy. Seitan is made of gluten, so people with celiac disease should avoid it. Tempeh and tofu are much easier to use and much healthier options.

There are many commercial meat-like substitutes. Choose wisely by looking for organic and non-GMO certified products, checking labels for minimally processed low or sodium, no dairy, no egg, no soy protein isolate, no starch, no isolated gluten, and minimal to no oil. If it contains only recognizable unprocessed plant ingredients, you can rest assured that will meet your health goal needs.

WHOLE GRAIN FLOUR AND REFINED FLOUR

"All-purpose" white flour is highly processed with most nutrients removed or stripped away, leaving only the starch. The nutrients have been used for making supplements, medications, vitamins, and other brand name high-priced products, so you should realize you are being robbed when you consume these expensive products. Many experts believe that if we replace refined white grains with whole grains, cancer rates will decrease by nearly 40 percent. These stripped grains are also a significant cause of countless cases of high blood pressure and high blood sugar in diabetes victims.

Whole grain (or whole wheat) flour is heavier and heartier and contains a lot of protein and fiber. Virtually anything you make with all-purpose flour can work with whole wheat flour instead. Try to lean toward the whole grains as much as possible. Once your taste buds adjust to them, you will find you will crave their nuttier, heartier flavor, though whole flour may be too dense for lighter cakes and pastries. In most recipes calling for white flour, you can often reduce whole grain flour by about 20 percent because it is quite absorptive and can make mixes very dense or you can use a whole grain pastry flour, spelt flour, or white whole wheat flour instead.

Whole grain pastry flour is lighter in color and weight and usually lower in protein and other nutrients. It typically works well for fluffier cakes, muffins, bread, and pastry recipes.

Brown rice flour and buckwheat flour is often used as the whole grain replacement flour for gluten-sensitive people. The darker brown rice flour contains more nutrients than whiter rice flour, just as whole wheat flours do, and it has a slightly nutty taste. Almond, bean, potato, spelt, and corn flour are used as substitutes by people with gluten sensitivities. Check labels for purity. Brown rice flour and buckwheat flour are good for baking heavier food like brownies, cookies, coffee cakes, and bread.

THICKENERS OTHER THAN REFINED CORNSTARCH AND FLOUR

Agar Powder or Flakes

Agar is a unique vegetable protein consisting of about 80 percent fiber derived from red or purple algae in seaweed. It comes in a white powder or flakes, is colorless, and odorless when heated with liquid. It must be heated for about five minutes to activate its thickening properties. It is used in place of gelatin to thicken soups, preserves, puddings, custards, meringue, Jell-O, and other desserts. When using it to thicken gravy or other liquid, the usual amount is 1 teaspoon agar to 1 cup of liquid, and for a Jell-O consistency, use about 1 ½ tablespoons of agar per cup of liquid.

Arrowroot Powder

Arrowroot powder is made from the root of a tropical tuber called the arrowroot plant. It is minimally processed and actually contains some fiber and protein, unlike white flour or cornstarch. Arrowroot powder is used in the same way in baking and for thickening sauces and gravy.

Xanthan Gum Powder

Xanthan gum absorbs water quickly, thickens, and stabilizes food at room temperature. It has been well-researched and is considered safe by the FDA to consume. It is used to thicken food and liquids for patients with swallowing difficulties. Xanthan gum has been shown to have the potential to help lower cholesterol and blood sugar levels.

Xanthan gum is commonly found in commercial food and frequently used as an egg replacement by vegans, though using crushed flaxseeds or unsweetened applesauce as "eggs" in baking are considered healthier options. Xanthan gum is highly resistant to freezing but is not the best at suppressing crystals in ice cream.

When adding xanthan gum, keep in mind that it tends to clump when not combined with dry ingredients first and should be spread out or dispersed evenly over liquids. Xanthan is another substance used to make jelled desserts, thicken gravy, and thicken or emulsify salad dressings. It is a good substitute for those with gluten allergies for adding structure and stickiness to gluten-free dough by adding 1 teaspoon for every cup of flour. As an oil substitute in your salad dressing, use 1/4 teaspoon xanthan per cup of liquid and a little more than 1/4 teaspoon per cup of a liquid consisting of a combination of water, juice, and vinegar. For jam consistency use 3/4 teaspoon per cup and for gelatin consistency use 1 ½ teaspoons.

Guar Gum

Guar gum is derived from seeds of the guar plant, which is a bean legume. It prevents crystallization in frozen ice cream and adds thickness to soups and nondairy products. Combine it with dry ingredients or blend well to prevent gummy clumping. It is activated at room temperature, but it takes about an hour to absorb. Like xanthan gum, guar gum contributes thickening, strength, and volume to baked goods, but does not provide as much elasticity. For this reason, xanthan gum is a better choice for yeast-based baked goods. Use a little more than 1/2 teaspoon of guar gum for every cup of flour.

WHOLE GRAINS, ANCIENT GRAINS, AND REFINED GRAINS

Whole grains such as whole wheat, whole rice, whole grain pasta, and whole-grain bread are an important source of complex carbohydrates, rich in nutrients, containing healthy phytoestrogen, B vitamins, iron, fiber, and antioxidants that help fight many diseases. Whole grains are typically darker in color due to their fiber coating, and white grains or refined grains have the fiber coating or bran removed. The highest-level whole grain consumers have consistently shown to have a lower risk of cardiovascular disease, type 2 diabetes, and cancer. Daily consumption of all three parts of whole grains appears to be as powerful as, and better than high blood pressure medication in alleviating hypertension[64]. The bran and germ layers in whole grains are the parts that are rich in fiber and nutrients. Whole grain consumption is generally related to higher satiety and a lower glycemic response when compared with refined grains[65]. Some ancient grains are becoming quite popular today. One is spelt, which is a type of wheat that contains gluten and works well for making bread, pasta, and baked goods. Bulgur (or cracked wheat) is a grain that comes in various sizes and cuts that can absorb flavor. It has a texture a lot like hamburger when used to make burgers, stews, soups, tacos, lasagna, casseroles, etc. Barley is a delicious, nutty, pasta-like grain that adds a lot of body and heartiness to soups and stews. Farro has a nutty flavor and chewy texture and a lot of fiber and can be substituted for brown rice or pasta and combined with tofu and veggies for a nutrient-dense meal.

About 75 percent of all whole grain produced worldwide is fed to animals. Most humans consume extraordinary amounts of refined or white grains stripped of their nutrients in the form of white rice, white flour, white pasta, and white bread. According to the US Dietary Guidelines, it is recommended that adults consume at least three ounces of *whole-grain* products daily. One slice of whole grain bread weighs about one ounce and contains about 69 calories. For the general population not consuming whole grains, more than 10,000 calories per day must be consumed in order to meet grain nutrient requirements. People who consume whole grains have much improved digestion, enhanced weight loss, and lower body mass indexes[66]. That's me! And can be you!

Gluten Allergy Whole Grain Alternatives

As discussed earlier in Chapter 12, people with celiac disease are allergic to gluten, which is found in particular grains like wheat, barley, and rye. Whole grains that are best suited for gluten allergy plant-based diets that are high in protein are quinoa, amaranth, and teff. Other healthy whole grains suitable for gluten allergies, though not as complete in protein nutrition are brown rice, millet and sorghum.

Popular Complete Protein Types and Their Use:

* Quinoa is a well-known complete protein that contains all nine essential amino acids. It is a gluten-free grain-like seed that is a member of the amaranth family, which includes spinach and chard. It is used in salads, served with roasted veggies, in bowls, as a side dish, and in stews.

* Amaranth is another complete protein containing the nine essential amino acids that will pair up with the other 11 made by the human body. It is similar to quinoa and is small, light tan, and used in similar ways as rice and oats. It can be eaten as a pilaf or porridge and is also ground into a gluten-free flour to be used in baking.

* Teff is the world's smallest grain and is packed with healthy nutrients and is yet another complete protein. It has an earthy, nutty flavor and lighter varieties tend to be slightly sweet. It has become quite popular as a super nutritious food and can be ground into a flour and used in baking in place of wheat flour, though it tends to be more expensive than other whole grains.

Brown Rice and White Rice (Gluten-Free)

Brown rice is a whole grain, meaning it contains all of its original three parts, including the germ, the bran, and the endosperm. With the germ and bran, brown rice is full of fiber and nutrient-rich. White rice is the remaining endosperm or starch after brown rice is stripped of its nutrients. Brown rice helps lower cholesterol, moves food through the digestive tract, relieves hunger, may help prevent the formation of blood clots, lowers the risk for certain cancers, and reduces the risk of heart disease, stroke, and type 2 diabetes. Long grain rice is higher in amylase, a digestive enzyme in our saliva that helps break down complex carbohydrates or starch, and short-grain rice is higher in amylopectin, a carbohydrate that is an insoluble form of starch, which makes it stickier. There are concerns about arsenic accumulating in the bran of rice, but to eliminate this concern, cook rice as you would cook pasta. Brown rice (and wild rice) should be prepared as follows: 1 cup of brown rice, simmered in 6 cups of water for 35 minutes, drain well, then cover with a lid let set on warm burner for about 15 minutes to steam and fluff. This process removes more than 50% of the potential arsenic content, bringing it down to a safe level for consumption.

Wild Rice

Wild rice is another whole grain from an aquatic grass containing many nutrients and health benefits. Native Americans grew it as a staple for hundreds of years. Wild rice contains slightly more protein than other whole rice grains and plenty of fiber.

All grains should at least be rinsed well, but it is recommended they are cooked as mentioned above to remove antinutrients and other potential contaminants. Use a fine-mesh strainer or cheesecloth for rinsing smaller sized seeds and grains. As stated above, grains such as brown rice should be cooked as you would cook pasta in 6 times as much water, then drained well to remove potential toxins (1 cup rice to 6 cups water).

Pasta

Use whole grain pasta, chickpea pasta, lentil pasta, or other vegetable pasta to replace white nonnutritive pasta. If using vegetable pasta, combine it with whole-grain bread for a fully nutritious and complete protein meal. When making sauces for food like spaghetti or lasagna, it is easy to incorporate greens, beans, and other vegetables to ensure that you and your family get a variety of nutritional benefits.

Chocolate and Cocoa

Cocoa and Cacao are virtually the same thing. The original plant is called a cacao plant. Cocoa or 100 percent powder ground from the beans of a cacao plant boasts many health benefits, thanks to its plethora of antioxidants, minerals, and fiber. It can improve cardiovascular health, reduce inflammation, boost the immune system, calm the nervous system, and protect against cancer. There is, however, an enormous difference between raw dark cocoa and the sugary, buttery chocolate concoctions you find in stores. The latter are typically loaded with sugar, oil, butter, artificial colors, and additives. Stick with 100 percent cocoa powder, and combine it with nondairy milk, banana, and vanilla for a sweet smoothie treat.

Whew!

So there you have it—a starter guide to help you stock your cupboards and fridge with remarkable ingredients to make excellent whole-food plant-based dishes. This lengthy list proves that the amazingly tasty, healthy dishes you can make will be endless. That, in itself, I hope, should excite you about embarking on your new journey to healthy living.

In Summary...

Wherever you are on your health journey, realize how unique *you* are. With all the information you now have, you should have a better understanding of how food affects you personally. Check your family history, know your health risks, what your body is capable of, and recognize your personal habits. For example, if blood pressure is an issue, avoid or reduce salt, meat, and processed food. If you want to lose weight, avoid fat, oil, meat, processed food, and alcohol. Want to prevent cancer, do all the above and certainly avoid eggs. It is not a one size fits all unless you want the ultimate health improvement experience overall with a better guarantee that you won't develop any health problems. In that case, apply all of the things you've learned. I guarantee your body will transform into an amazing fuel burning machine!

You have more control than you realize to reroute your destiny, improve your life, and be happy simply by making sure that you eat the most natural and healthiest food on earth. Why spend the last half or third of your life taking medications that have side effects that drag you down, make you feel tired and miserable, living your life battling against diseases that control you? Get up, get out, take control, enjoy a whole food plant-based diet, and love yourself and your life.

You can do it.

   You won't regret it.

      I guarantee it!

         Now let's get cooking!

Cookbook
Recipes for Life

While spending nearly thirty years with military spouses from a variety of cultural backgrounds, acknowledging that we shared a primary focus on our children's health and happiness, we also realized that food gatherings stood out as a common thread that bound us together. These gatherings kept us going in positive directions while our spouses were deployed to dangerous regions around the world. Many in our close groups were, and still are, health-conscious personal trainers, dancers, nutritionists, nurses, health writers, and so on. We grew close relationships and created cookbooks containing sweet memories of our time spent together. Knowing that food brings such comfort and togetherness, rather than giving up food that was unhealthy, I took on the challenge of converting it to plant-based versions with a primary focus on health and healing to share with family, friends, and my patients. I will now share some of these recipes with you.

GETTING ORGANIZED– VERY IMPORTANT

I am a spice lover! I can't deny it. I pride myself on using healthy, natural medicinal gifts from nature to season our meals and increase the variety of nutrients for optimizing health.

Once you've acquired some of your staples and your first week's meal plan and ingredients, clear out the cabinets and refrigerator of any nonplant food. Plenty of places like churches and shelters will welcome canned food and unopened packaged food for those in need. It is such a great feeling to start fresh and new. The goal is to make cooking exciting, simple, fun, colorful, healthy, and delicious!

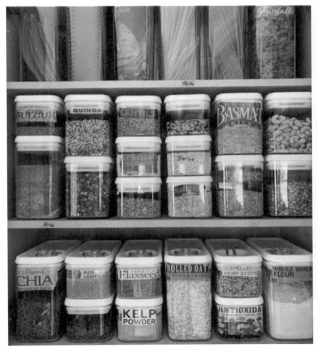
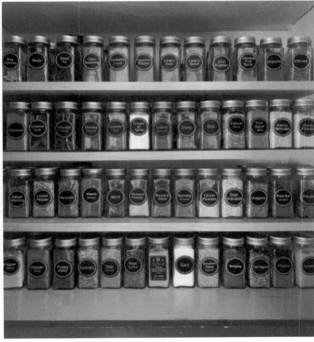

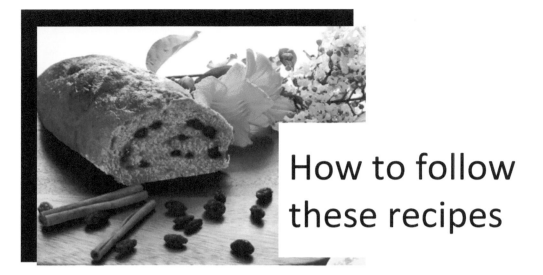

How to follow these recipes

SERVING SIZES:

The majority of these recipes are designed for serving sizes of 4 to 5 people. Some recipes are designed as large batches for freezing leftovers such as the megahealthy Daily Dozen Spaghetti, chili, and some stews.

* Begin by doing two of any of these: Give up fried food. Replace white breads with *whole* grain breads and grains. Replace eggs in your baked goods with flax "egg" gel. Replace butter in your cookies and brownies with whole puréed avocado, nut, or seed butters. Replace white sugar with anything from the substitute chart. Find a plant-based milk you can enjoy. Just doing two of these results in a quick ten-pound weight loss. Pounds will literally melt away.

* Ingredients with multiple options are listed in order from healthiest and most practical to less healthy when possible. You can use the tastier alternatives for early taste bud conversion to gently bring around picky eaters.

  Example: date paste, date syrup, molasses, honey, maple syrup or pure cane sugar, in that order, from the healthiest to the least healthy. Date sugar, date paste, molasses, and fruit are the healthiest sweeteners/sugars. Then pure honey and maple, in that order have some nutritional value. Cane sugar has very little nutritive value, but sometimes it works well for consistency and can be mixed with date sugar.

* Alternative ingredients, like tahini/sesame seed butter, hemp seed butter, pumpkin seed butter, potatoes, and cauliflower, are listed for allergy sensitive individuals. The term "whole grain," as discussed in the section on gluten sensitivities is a flexible term for whole wheat replacements.

  Many ingredients can easily be swapped out to accommodate gluten sensitivity health needs like brown rice, buckwheat, teff, and millet.

* Note: Recipe titles and ingredients in "quotes" are plant-based representations of animal-based products. For example, a recipe with the taste, texture, and appearance of bacon or egg that is made from all plant-based ingredients may be referred to as "bacon," "parmesan cheese," "mayonnaise," or "egg". These quoted titles are meant to help you find recipes easier.

* I reference "organic" or "vegan" ingredients especially when it comes to commercially prepared sauces like ketchup, tortillas, and Worcestershire sauce mostly because buying organic or vegan helps you avoid ingredients such as high fructose corn syrup, lard, and anchovies.

* Remember that variety is the key for acquiring all of the health benefits and complete nutrition a whole food plant-based diet offers. Of equal importance is to limit the amount of plant food containing high amounts of fat such as coconut, avocado, nuts, and olives. Consume limited amounts of sweet plant food such as maple syrup, honey, pineapple, dates, date sugar, and raisins. Limit intake of salty food and try to remember to buffer such food with soy products.

* There is really no need to track nutritional data for recipes when you follow these simple rules because you will have achieved the highest level of health possible.

* The following recipes will help you avoid un-healthy, processed food and chemical additives, and my hope is that more companies will commit to using natural plant food sources to preserve, color, and add texture to commercially prepared food in stores and restaurants everywhere one day soon.

*You are about to encounter some recipes that have been converted using the principles you've just learned. Throughout the first half of this book, I have shared numerous sites that offer plenty of other Whole Food, Plant-Based recipes. You now have the tools to replace any unhealthy ingredient in any recipe, and any improvement in your diet with plant-based food will very likely make a noticeable difference in your health, the way you feel,
and in your appearance.*

Enjoy your new lease on life!

Kitchen Tools You Will Likely Need

There is no need to go out and buy all of the supplies and ingredients for a plant-based lifestyle right away. Acquire a little at a time. Enjoy as you learn a new way of recreating your own healthy recipes.

Food processor or vegetable chopper

Blender or high-powered mixer

Rubber spatula

Fine mesh strainer and regular colander or strainer

Sharp knives and cutting boards

Measuring spoons, measuring cups, and mixing bowls

Nonstick skillets—if coated, they should be intact and used with controlled heat (medium heat or lower)

Saucepans and pots

Mini coffee grinder

Finding Your New Ingredients

You will become familiar with many natural ingredient alternatives and until the industries, restaurants, and grocery stores become more familiar with carrying them, they may be somewhat difficult to find. But don't fret, they aren't as hard to find as you may think. Several stores are now carrying many plant-based food items. Currently, Whole Foods and Trader Joes seem to be in the lead. Anything you can't find in your local grocery store you can order online. Here is a list to help you get started.

Tofu and Tempeh are usually found in the refrigerated section near the nondairy products.

Miso paste is usually found in the refrigerated section near tofu, tempeh, and other nondairy products. It may also be found in health food aisle near peanut butter and condiments or in the international food aisle.

Tahini is often found near the peanut butter and other nut butters or in the international food aisle. You can also make your own.

Flaxseed is usually found in the health food aisle near other seeds like chia seeds. Best to buy them whole and crush yourself for optional nutrient value.

Nutritional Yeast or Nooch is usually found in the baking goods aisle near baker's yeast.

Date Sugar is usually found in the baking goods aisle and fresh dates are found in the produce department. Dried dates can also be found with dried fruit such as raisins, pineapple, bananas, etc.

Dates are usually found in the produce section and date paste can be made from them.
Seaweed is usually found in the International food aisle and in Asian markets.

Xanthan Gum or Agar is usually found in the health food or spices aisle.

Seasonings, Herbs, and Spices

Salt Reduction Seasoning Blend

Chickenless Bouillon Powder

Nutritional Oil

Vegetable Stock

Taco Seasoning

Mushroom Stock

Beefless Bouillon

Soybean Powder

Italian Seasoning

Seafood Seasoning

Date Paste and Date Syrup

Umami or Worcestershire Sauce

Salt Reduction Seasoning Spice Blend

This seasoning quickly adds flavor, has sweet and salty tones that make your taste buds happy, spices that have been shown to reduce cancer and inflammation and soothe anxiety. Soy powder helps reduce the damaging effects of salt and kelp helps ensure you get the iodine you may need since many people now use non-iodized sea salt. Add this blend to a shaker and place it on your table to grab in place of salt.

INGREDIENTS
1 tablespoon dried basil
1 tablespoon garlic powder
1 tablespoon parsley flakes
1 tablespoon nutritional yeast
1-2 teaspoons ground black pepper
2 teaspoons onion powder
1/2 - 1 teaspoon natural salt, adjust to taste/health
1 1/2 teaspoons soy powder/dried soybean
   (See recipe)

1 teaspoon celery seed
1/2 teaspoon coriander
1/2 teaspoon turmeric
1/4 teaspoon kelp powder
1/8 - 1/4 teaspoon cayenne pepper

PREPARATION
Combine all ingredients and place in a shaker to
   add nutrients and flavor to any meal.

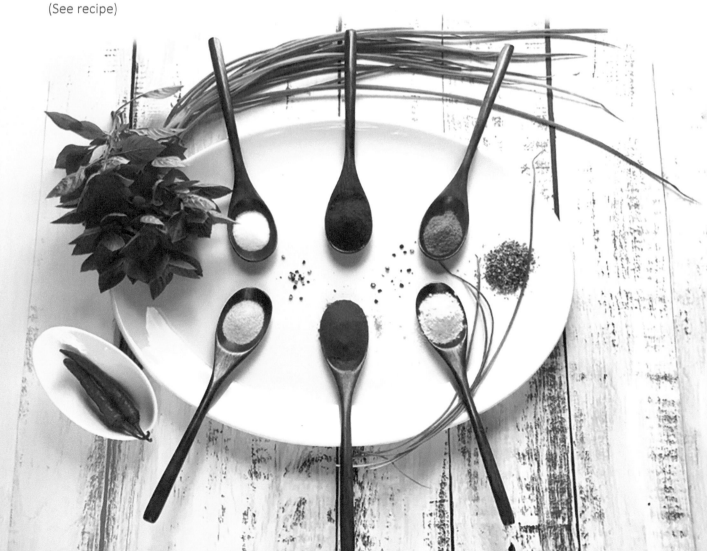

Chickenless Bouillon Powder

Spices help trick your taste buds into not missing the salt. This bouillon is significantly lower in the damaging effects of table salt that can cause hypertension and cancer.

INGREDIENTS

1/2 cup nutritional yeast
2 teaspoons onion powder
1/4 teaspoon turmeric
3/4 teaspoon Italian seasoning
1 teaspoon dried parsley
1 teaspoon garlic powder
1/4 teaspoon celery seed
1/2 teaspoon dried sage
1/4 teaspoon dried thyme

1/2 - 1 teaspoon natural salt, adjust to taste/health
1 teaspoon soy powder to help buffer salt (See recipe)
1/8 teaspoon fresh ground pepper

PREPARATION

* Add all ingredients to a blender and pulse to blend to a powder.
* For broth, use 1 tablespoon vegetable or chickenless bouillon powder per 1 cup hot water. (Consider using miso paste for additional salt flavoring in soup or gravy after cooking it).

Nutritional Oil

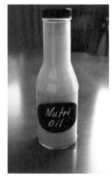

Many people say, "I could never give up oil". I was once one of those people. Olives contain some oil and many people believe that olive oil is healthy. The process that most olives go through to make enough oil for the population not only removes all or nearly all of the nutrients, including the important cholesterol-removing fiber, but chemicals are added as well. Some chemicals are used to separate the oil from the fruit and other chemicals are added as well, resulting in a less than healthy substance. See supporting science and information under 'Omega Sources to Avoid'. As stated earlier, replacing or avoiding oil is especially important for those with cholesterol issues and weight gain concerns. Chemicals are a concern with regard to cancer and the imbalanced omegas, even in extra virgin olive oil can cause other inflammatory diseases as well. Make a double batch of this much healthier version of oil each week for making your own homemade salad dressings and remember to use it in other recipes that call for oil as well. You will lose weight and your cholesterol levels will fall. This oil replacement can be stored in the refrigerator for a week or so.

INGREDIENTS

1 cup warm water
1 teaspoon nutritional yeast, to taste
1 teaspoon light miso paste

THICKENING INGREDIENT OPTIONS

1/4 teaspoon xanthan powder, 2 teaspoons crushed flaxseed, or 1-2 teaspoons tahini, optional
  (xanthan powder and flaxseed take 5-10 minutes to thicken)

PREPARATION

Add ingredients to a blender and blend well for 30 seconds to a minute until smooth.
The tahini or flaxseed mixture will be a bit cloudy compared to oil.

Vegetable Stock (Broth)

This is a healthy staple to use in place of cooking oil for adding moisture when sautéing food. It can also be used when preparing grains, pasta, soups, and stews in place of water to provide additional nutrients.

INGREDIENTS

2 cups onion, red and yellow, roughly chopped, add to food processor
1 cup of carrot, roughly chopped, add to food processor
2 ribs of celery, roughly chopped, add to food processor
2-3 cloves of garlic, roughly chopped, add to food processor
1/2 cup fresh or moistened mushrooms or 1 tablespoon dried mushroom powder (porcini, portobello, and/or shiitake preferred)
1/3 cup fresh parsley, kale, and/or spinach, chopped or 2 tablespoons dried parsley
1/2 teaspoon fresh ground black pepper
1 tablespoon nutritional yeast (usually found in the baking section near conventional yeast)
2 tablespoons light miso paste or 1 tablespoon low sodium soy sauce

PREPARATION

* Add all the ingredients except for nutritional yeast and miso or soy sauce to a food processor to finely mince, then transfer everything to a large nonstick pot.

* Simmer over medium heat for about 30 minutes until caramelized or lightly browned. Use a small amount of water, if needed to keep it moist.

* Add 6-7 cups of water, bring to short boil, reduce heat to simmer, and cook for an hour or so.

* Allow broth to cool for about 20 minutes, then add nutritional yeast, and soy sauce or miso.

* Blend with either an immersion blender or transfer to a blender for a smoother consistency.

* Transfer stock to jars or containers with a good seal. Use within 10 days in the refrigerator or within a couple months if frozen. You can add miso or soy after boiling and follow canning directions for storage.

Taco Seasoning

On busy evenings, taco seasoning is great to have on hand for whipping up quick, healthy tacos using whatever vegetables you have on hand in your refrigerator.

INGREDIENTS
1/4 cup hot chili powder
3 tablespoons paprika
1 tablespoon ground cumin
2 tablespoons onion powder
1 tablespoon nutritional yeast
1 tablespoon garlic powder
1 tablespoon oregano
1 1/2 teaspoons black pepper
1/4 teaspoon cayenne pepper

1-3 teaspoons salt, optional, to taste/health
1 tablespoon organic soy powder to help
   buffer salt (See recipe)

PREPARATION
Combine all ingredients.
Label and save as a spice.
See *Lentil Tempeh Taco Wraps*, find a recipe online, or create your own.

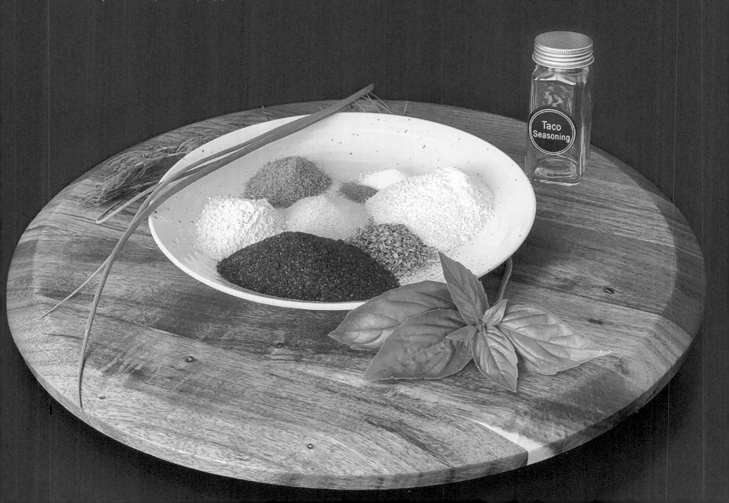

Mushroom Stock (Broth)

Mushroom stock has a meatier flavor, and is especially useful for making darker, more beeflike gravy and stews.

INGREDIENTS

1 1/2 cups yellow onion, roughly chopped or sliced
2 cups mushrooms, roughly chopped or sliced
3 cloves garlic, sliced
2 celery ribs, roughly chopped or sliced
2 tablespoons dried porcini mushrooms soaked in 1/2 cup hot vegetable broth or water for 20-30 minutes
1/2 teaspoon dried sage
1/4 teaspoon kelp powder or 2 teaspoons crushed nori seaweed
1/4 teaspoon black pepper
1 tablespoon miso paste or low sodium soy sauce
5 cups vegetable stock, broth, or water, adjust as desired

PREPARATION

* Simmer onion in a nonstick pot over medium heat for 30 minutes to caramelize.

* Add mushrooms, garlic, and celery and cook another 10 minutes until tender.

* Allow to cool enough to safely transfer to a blender, add remaining ingredients, except miso or low sodium soy sauce, and add just enough broth or water to blend to a purée.

* Transfer back to pot, add desired amount of vegetable broth or water, and simmer on low for 6-8 hours.

* Allow it to cool for about 20 minutes, then add miso or soy sauce.

* Transfer stock to jars or containers with a good seal, place in the refrigerator, and use within 10 days or within a couple months if frozen.

Beefless Bouillon Powder

INGREDIENTS

3-4 dried shiitake or porcini mushrooms for powdered bouillon
  (or use fresh mushrooms, 1/2 cup + 1/2 cup water for quick use)
1 teaspoon garlic powder
1 teaspoon onion powder
1/2 teaspoon cocoa powder
1/2 teaspoon coriander
1/2 teaspoon paprika
3/4 teaspoon black pepper
2 bay leaves, break off stems
3-4 tablespoons dark miso

PREPARATION

Add ingredients to a blender or to a coffee grinder and blend to a powder/paste.

Soybean Powder

Soybeans are a member of the legume family. They are complete proteins, loaded with heart-healthy fiber, iron, potassium, and isoflavone phytonutrients that protect us against many forms of cancer. Soybeans help reduce the damaging effects of salt on our blood vessels, thereby reducing hypertension. Add this powder to any dry food recipe containing salt/sodium, though continue to keep salt intake to a minimum or eliminate it entirely. Use fresh soybeans in other recipes when possible. Making soybean powder at home is easy. A thoroughly dry baked batch of of soybeans can last for many months in an airtight container.

INGREDIENTS

2-3 cups Fresh Edamame (ready-to-eat immature green soybeans removed from pods are mild in flavor and low in lectins)
    or use:
2-3 cups Dried soybeans (adult soybeans, high in lectin and saponins, must be soaked, rinsed, and boiled)
Note: In low amounts, lectins are protective and beneficial to humans. High levels can cause digestive problems.

PREPARATION

* Dehydrate or bake fresh edamame (baby soybeans) on very low heat in the oven at 170°F for 8-10 hours, until dry.

* For commercially prepared, dried adult soybeans, boil, soak, and rinse them thoroughly before baking. They need to be boiled and soaked for 12 hours, rinsing them every few hours to remove excess lectins, saponins, and bitter flavor.

* After soybeans are dried, blend them into a powder using a coffee bean grinder, spread it out on a baking mat, place in oven for about 10-30 minutes more to ensure dryness. Cool and store soybean powder in an airtight container.

Italian Seasoning

This is a combination of herbs commonly used in Italian dishes, especially spaghetti and lasagna. It may be hard to find it in some locations but is easy enough to make yourself. Italian seasoning adds megaflavor and nutrients.

INGREDIENTS

2 tablespoons basil, dried
2 tablespoons oregano, dried
1 tablespoon garlic powder
1 tablespoon thyme, dried
1 tablespoon rosemary, dried
2 teaspoons sage, dried

PREPARATION

Mix all ingredients. Label and save as a spice.

"Seafood" Seasoning (Old Bay)

Raised near Annapolis, Maryland, my family regularly entertained guests with bushels of Maryland Blue Crabs seasoned with Old Bay, a popular classic from Baltimore. This recipe reduces the amount of salt and is a very tasty addition to plant-based seafood flavored meals.

INGREDIENTS
1 bay leaf, dried
1 tablespoon celery seed
1 teaspoon natural salt, to taste/health
1 teaspoon soy powder to help buffer salt (See recipe)
1 tablespoon dark miso
2 teaspoons smoked or regular paprika
1/4 teaspoon red pepper flakes
1/2 teaspoon black pepper
1/8 teaspoon dry mustard
1 teaspoon seaweed (Wakame, dulse, Nori, Alaria) or 1/8 teaspoon kelp powder

PREPARATION
Blend into a powder using a coffee bean grinder and store in an airtight container as a spice.

Date Paste and Date Syrup

This sweetener is quite healthy due to its abundance of antioxidants and fiber. Dates have a glycemic index of about 49, a little lower than maple syrup at 54, and much lower than white sugar at 100. These numbers show how whole forms of sweeteners can have a much lower impact on blood sugar levels than processed sugar. Processed sugar spikes and can be very dangerous, especially for diabetics. Date paste is cloudy in its purest form as it contains a lot of fiber. For more syrup-like consistency, date paste can be heated with a little more water added and cheesecloth can be used to remove some of the fiber but try not to go overboard. That fiber is very important :0)

INGREDIENTS
1 cup of pitted dates
1 cup of water (1/2 cup for date paste)

PREPARATION
* Add dates and water to a saucepan, cover, bring to a short boil, stir, remove from heat, and allow to cool.

* Transfer to a blender, and blend until smooth and syrupy.

* Consider adding a little lemon for some zing, 1-2 teaspoons.

Umami Sauce

Adapted from Dr. Michael Greger and found in his *How Not to Die Cookbook*, this sauce will help you cut down on salt levels in soy sauce and it tastes similar to Worcestershire sauce. Umami sauce was developed by a Japanese chemist—a delicious flavor designed to appeal to all of your taste buds.

INGREDIENTS

1 cup low sodium vegetable broth, nutritional oil, or water (see nutritional oil recipe)
1 teaspoon garlic, minced
1 teaspoon fresh ginger, minced or 1/4 teaspoon garlic powder
1 tablespoon blackstrap molasses
1 ½ teaspoons date syrup or date sugar
1/2 teaspoon tomato paste
1/2 teaspoon ground black pepper
1 ½ teaspoons light miso paste blended with 2 tablespoons water (slurry)
2 teaspoons blended peeled lemon
1 tablespoon rice vinegar

PREPARATION

Combine all ingredients, except for miso, lemon, and vinegar in a saucepan over medium heat and bring to a simmer for 3 minutes, then remove from heat. Allow to cool for a few minutes, then add remaining ingredients. Save in a jar or bottle with a lid in the refrigerator.

Breakfast Options

Pancakes

Southwest Eggy Burritos

Hash Brown Potatoes

Tempeh or Portobello Bacon

Oatmeal, All Season

Granola

Aussie Omega Protein Bites

Yogurt

Healthy food groups that people often miss out on are nuts, seeds, and fruit. Eating breakfast is a great way to ensure that you get many of the nutrients you need for a healthy body that you don't normally get throughout the remainder of the day.

Some popular, healthy, plant-based breakfast ideas are:

* Whole grain toast with avocado and any variation of onion, cilantro, jalapenos, tomatoes, basil, sprouts, capers, crushed flax or black pepper, along with a glass of fresh blended whole fruit juice or a smoothie.

* Whole grain bread with peanut or almond butter or seed butters made from sunflower, sesame, or pumpkin seed sprinkled with crushed flax, banana, honey, or maple syrup.

* Smoothies with berries, banana, dark leafy greens, flax, nondairy milk, nuts and/or seeds.

* Cinnamon pancakes with crushed flax blueberries and pure maple syrup, apple cinnamon raisin pancakes, or lemon chia pancakes.

* Oatmeal with any variation of nuts or seeds: walnuts, almonds, flax, pumpkin, chia or hemp. Fruit or berries: frozen, dried, or fresh including bananas, raisins, blueberries, strawberries, mangos, melons, cherries, or apricots. Top with granola, cinnamon, coconut flakes, maple syrup, or honey. Keep a variety of items on hand in airtight containers and set them out along with bowls of fresh fruit at breakfast for a really fun, fast, and easy way for everyone to create their own masterpiece. Most WFPB nutritional scientists say they eat oatmeal for breakfast every day. Oats with flax are incredibly nutritious and can lower blood sugar levels and reduce the risk of heart disease. Weight loss is commonly experienced while consuming oatmeal on a regular basis.

* Scrambled tofu "eggs" are so delicious that even an egg lover can be fooled by them. Sauté some sliced onions and bell peppers and add some seasonings. Make "bacon" ahead of time with tempeh, tofu, or portobello mushrooms. Consider making hash browns and add a side of fresh fruit as well. This is a masterpiece of a breakfast!

* Whole grain cereal or granola with nondairy milk. Use nondairy almond, soy, oat milk, or any other variety. If you combine two different milks, the flavors seem to meld and neutralize without a distinctive taste of either one. Almond milk is a very popular choice.

* Aussie Bites are an easy, healthy, and delicious treat for the family to grab on the go.

Pancakes with Berries or Apple Cinnamon Raisin

Weekends are a great time for the family to enjoy pancakes. Selections of nondairy milk for pancakes can make a big difference in texture, density, and stickiness. Oat milk works well for fluffier pancakes, soy milk and coconut milk make them denser and stickier, and almond milk makes them pastier. The type of flour makes a difference as well. Avoid almond flour in this recipe as it makes pancakes sticky and be patient - allow them to cook before flipping.

DRY MIX INGREDIENTS
1 cup whole grain flour
2 tablespoons date sugar
1 teaspoons baking powder
1/2 teaspoon baking soda
1/4 teaspoon cinnamon

WET MIX INGREDIENTS
1 tablespoon flaxseeds, crushed (to soak/gel in the following ingredients)
1 1/2 cups nondairy milk (we usually use both almond and soy milk)
1 teaspoon lemon juice
1/4 teaspoon salt + 1 teaspoon soy powder
1 teaspoon vanilla bean powder or extract

PREPARATION
* Preheat an intact nonstick skillet or griddle over medium heat for a few minutes before pouring in the pancake mix to help prevent sticking. No oil needed.
* Combine DRY MIX INGREDIENTS in a large measuring cup (4 cups) or bowl.
* In a separate pitcher or bowl, combine WET MIX INGREDIENTS.
* Combine wet and dry mixes. Allow to sit for at least 5 minutes, then press lumps against the sides with a spoon or fork to break them apart. Overstirring flattens pancakes.
* Allow pancakes to cook until some bubbles to form in the middle and the edges become a bit dry before flipping. If cooking for a large group, set oven on warm and place a plate with parchment paper on it to keep cooked pancakes warm until serving.
* Top with pure maple syrup, blueberry sauce (See recipe), fruit compote, or apple topping.

Blueberry Pancake Sauce

INGREDIENTS
1 cup blueberries, fresh or frozen
¼ cup pure maple syrup or date syrup
1 teaspoon lemon juice, optional for tartness
1 teaspoon whole grain flour or ¼ teaspoon xanthan gum

PREPARATION
* Place ingredients in a small saucepan over medium heat, stir to mix, and heat until slightly bubbly.
* Spoon blueberry sauce over pancakes.

Apple Cinnamon Raisin Pancake Topper

INGREDIENTS

2 apples, cubed

2 tablespoons water

1/2 cup raisins

1/4-1/2 teaspoon cinnamon

1/4 cup maple syrup or date syrup

1 teaspoon whole grain flour or 1/4 teaspoon agar or xanthan powder for thickening

PREPARATION Place apples and water in a saucepan over medium heat. Cover and heat for 10-15 minutes until apples are softened. Add remaining ingredients, and simmer uncovered

until desired consistency achieved.

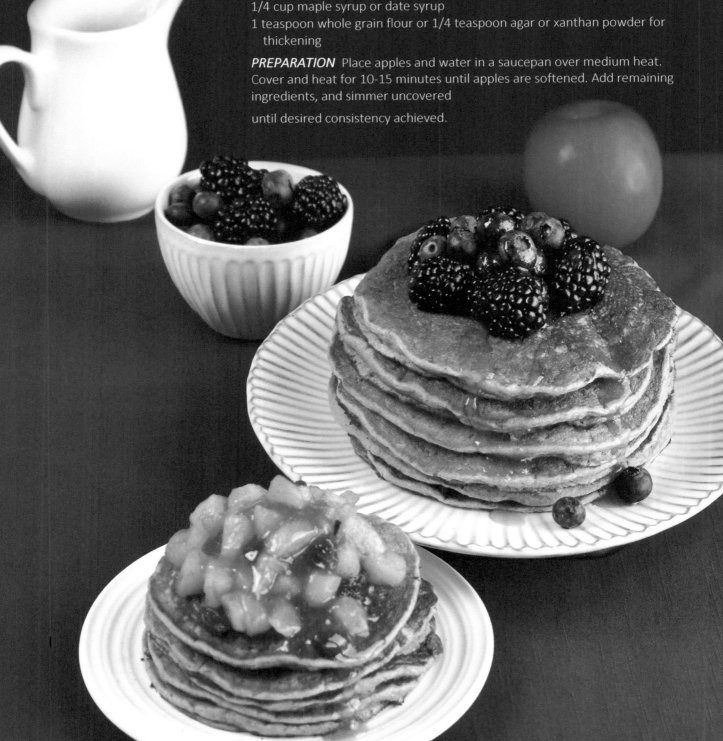

Scrambled Tofu Egg Burritos

Prefrozen silken tofu makes a great egg-like texture. Unfrozen firm tofu can also be used. Impress your guests with this healthy delicious breakfast, served with all the fixings of breakfast burritos - buffet style.

VEGETABLE SAUTÉ INGREDIENTS

1 cup onions, sliced
1 cup bell peppers or zucchini, sliced
1 cup leafy greens, mushrooms, or tomatoes, sliced or chopped
1/2 cup beans, optional
3 cloves garlic, minced/sliced or 1/4 teaspoon garlic powder
1 1/2 teaspoon cumin
1 1/2 teaspoon chili powder

SCRAMBLED TOFU "EGGS"

1 1/2 blocks of silken tofu (14-ounce blocks), frozen, thawed, and pressed to remove water (tofu shrinks in size when water is removed)
1-2 tablespoons light miso paste slurry (mixed with 2 tablespoon of warm water)
1/2 teaspoon kala namak (black salt) egg-flavored seasoning, divided
1/2 teaspoon turmeric, divided
2 tablespoons nutritional yeast

GARNISH AND SIDES

Self-serve buffet style with tortillas or toast, avocado, jalapeño peppers, salsa, cilantro, plant-based cheddar, sour cream, or bacon (tempeh bacon shown). And don't forget a bowl of mixed fruit!

PREPARATION

* Set up two nonstick skillets, one for the veggies and one for the tofu "eggs."

* Add VEGETABLE SAUTÉ INGREDIENTS to one of the skillets and use low sodium broth or water to keep moist—no oil needed. Sauté to desired crispiness or tenderness.

* In the other nonstick skillet over medium heat, add crumbled tofu and sprinkle with half of the turmeric and kala namak, then toss to mix and sprinkle the remaining half over tofu to coat evenly.

* Pour miso slurry over tofu, sprinkle with nutritional yeast, toss to combine, and heat through.

Hash Brown Potatoes

Enjoy these tasty toasty taters. These can be made into patties or into an omelet-like wrap filled with tofu scrambled "egg" and sautéed vegetables.

INGREDIENTS

3 medium potatoes, grated or shredded
1/2 cup mild onion, sliced thin or chopped and mixed with potato shreds, optional
2 teaspoons nutritional yeast
1-2 garlic cloves, minced, or 1/4 teaspoon garlic powder
1 tablespoon miso or 1/4 teaspoon salt + 1/2 teaspoon soy powder or soybeans, or serve with tofu eggs
¼ teaspoon black pepper, fresh ground to taste

PREPARATION

* In a bowl, combine shredded potatoes, onions, nutritional yeast, garlic, salt, and soy powder.

* Gently press and form shredded potato mix into 3/4-inch patties in a nonstick skillet to cook over medium heat, covered with a lid. Avoid adding water and overcooking to prevent mushiness.

* Check for doneness by lifting edge. It should take about 6-7 minutes on each side for some browning to occur.

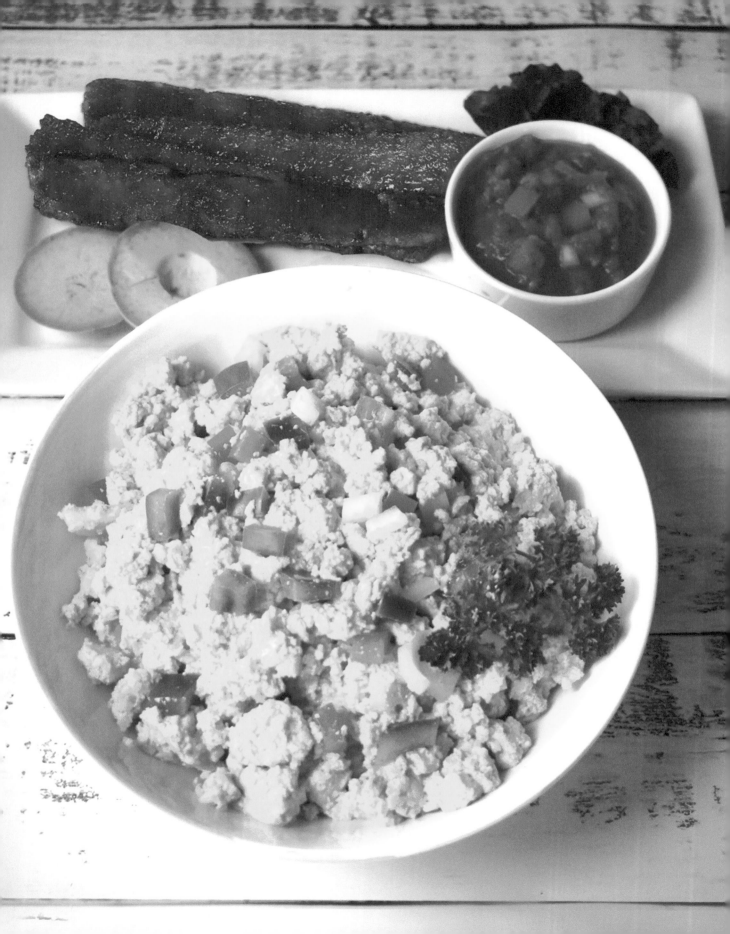

Tempeh or Portobello Bacon

Many people say they can't live without bacon, and I have to admit I had been one of them. This nonanimal bacon is much healthier than the traditional animal bacon. By comparison, it has no saturated fat, very low salt, no animal protein, or chemicals and contains incredible nutrients. It can be added to salads, enjoyed with scrambled "eggs," omelets, in BLTs (bacon, lettuce, and tomato) or other sandwiches, in wraps, on pasta dishes, and more. Make a large batch and marinate extra "bacon" to freeze and enjoy later. Portobello mushrooms and tempeh should be marinated for several hours or overnight to soak in the flavors. Super delicious and typically doesn't cause a heart attack!

"BACON" OPTIONS
One block (8 ounces) tempeh, 1/2 block (7 ounces) firm tofu, previously frozen, thawed, and pressed, or 2 large portobello mushrooms, thinly sliced into 1/4 inch strips. Marinate tempeh for about and hour and mushrooms for at least 6 hours for richer flavor.

MARINADE INGREDIENTS
1/4 cup nutritional oil (See recipe)
1/4 cup maple syrup
2 tablespoon nutritional yeast
1/2 teaspoon garlic powder
1 teaspoon ground black pepper
2 teaspoon smoked paprika
2 teaspoon liquid smoke
1/4 cup low sodium soy sauce or tamari, to taste/health

PREPARATION

* Mix together MARINADE INGREDIENTS in a medium bowl or dish. If using tempeh or mushroom strips soak them for at least 30 minutes to an hour or so.

* Preheat oven to 350°F.

* Prepare a nonstick baking mat or parchment paper lined baking sheet.

* Transfer strips to the baking mat or parchment paper and bake for about 15 minutes until strips are caramelized and somewhat crispy on the outside. Keep an eye on them to prevent burning.

* For crispier "bacon," gently turn them over, baste with more marinade, and bake for another 15-20 minutes, watching them closely.

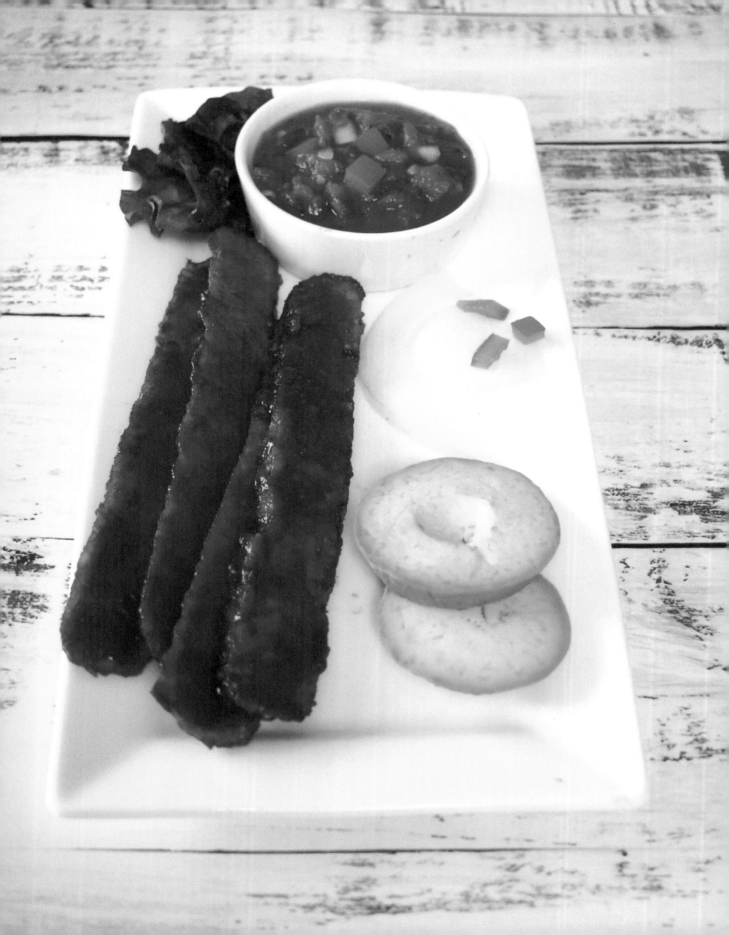

Oatmeal for all Seasons

Top nutritional scientists will tell you that making oatmeal a regular habit is one of the best, if not the best thing you can do for cardiac health. It is high in fiber, a great way to incorporate flaxseed, chia seeds, hempseeds, fruit, nuts, and spices. You can avoid making your hot oatmeal gooey by heating the milk separately to enjoy in the winter or soak it overnight with cold milk in the refrigerator for summer enjoyment. Add a handful nuts, coconut, or raisins and banana slices.

INGREDIENTS
1 cup rolled oats
1 tablespoon flaxseeds, pumpkin seeds, or chia seeds
1/2 teaspoon cinnamon
1 1/2 -2 cups nondairy milk
1-2 tablespoons date syrup, date sugar, honey, or maple syrup
1/2 teaspoon vanilla bean powder, paste, or extract
1 cup mixed berries and fruit, fresh or frozen (add when ready to eat)

PREPARATION
For overnight oatmeal, combine first six ingredients in a bowl and place them in the refrigerator.

Granola

Granola is very easy to make at home and for a fraction of the cost. You can tweak this with various spices and try using other whole grains such as spelt, barley, or wheat.

INGREDIENTS
3 cups rolled oats
1/4 cup flaxseed, ground
1/4 cup pumpkin seeds
1/3 cup date sugar
1/4 cup date syrup, honey, or maple syrup
2 tablespoons water
1 1/2 teaspoon cinnamon
1 tablespoon dark miso paste
1/4 teaspoon baking soda
1 teaspoon vanilla bean powder, paste, or extract
1/4 cup raisins, blueberries, or other fruit
1/4 cup raw walnuts or pecans, coarsely chopped, optional

PREPARATION
* Preheat oven to 300°F.
* Prepare a large baking sheet lined with parchment paper or a baking mat.
* Combine the oats, flaxseeds, and pumpkin seeds in a large bowl.

* In a saucepan, combine sugar, syrup/honey, and water and stir while bringing to a controlled boil for about a minute. Remove from heat and allow to cool for 5 minutes.
* Add miso and vanilla to the saucepan, combine cinnamon and baking soda and add to the saucepan, and stir and pour over the oats and seeds. Toss to coat.
* Spread the mixture out in a thin layer on the baking mat or parchment paper. Bake for 15 minutes, then stir and flip over and bake for another 15 minutes until lightly browned, watching closely to prevent burning.
* Remove from the oven, add the fruit, nuts, or additional seeds to the baking sheet, toss to combine and break apart into pieces when cool enough to handle. It will harden as it cools to room temperature.
* Serve over yogurt with fruit or fruit compote, as a cereal with milk, on ice cream or on toast with peanut butter and banana.

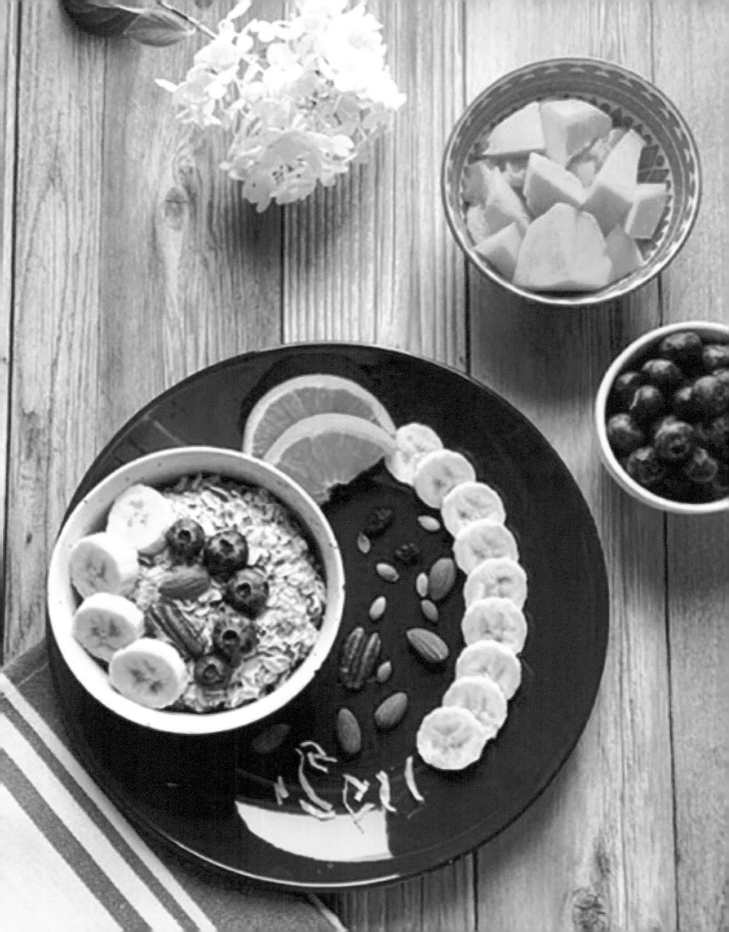

Super Healthy "Aussie Bites"

A good friend introduced me to "Aussie Bites" several years ago. We loved them so much we had to find a way to recreate these little lovelies at home without oil or milk. Depending on what you have on hand they can vary in flavor, but they are always a delicious treat. These can be reshaped into protein snack bars (less bake time for thinner shapes).

INGREDIENTS

2 cups oats, divided (1 cup powdered)

2 dates, slice around midsection, flip lid and
   remove seed

1 banana, cut up in chunks

1 ½ - 2 cups dried apricots

1/4 cup ground flaxseed

1/4 cup shredded coconut, nuts, or hemp seeds

1/4 cup quinoa, rinsed and uncooked

1/2 teaspoon cinnamon

1/4 teaspoon baking soda

1/4 cup hempseeds or sunflower seeds

1/4 cup pumpkin seeds

1/4 cup nut or seed butter (tahini), avocado, or
   applesauce

2-4 tablespoons honey, date syrup, or pure
   maple syrup

1/2 teaspoon vanilla bean powder, vanilla paste,
   or extract

2 tablespoons chia seeds

PREPARATION

* Preheat oven to 350°F.

* Pour 1 cup of oats into a food processor and blend for about 30 seconds. Add second cup of oats along with all remaining ingredients, and pulse gently until chopped into small pieces.

* Fill 1 ½ inch diameter fleximold or nonstick muffin cups about 3/4 full without packing them too tight or do the same with larger cups. You could also roll a tablespoon of these up in a ball in your hands to bake on a baking mat.

* Bake in the preheated oven for about 9 minutes until lightly browned or up to 15 minutes longer w/larger cups. Allow them to cool a bit before removing from the muffin cups.

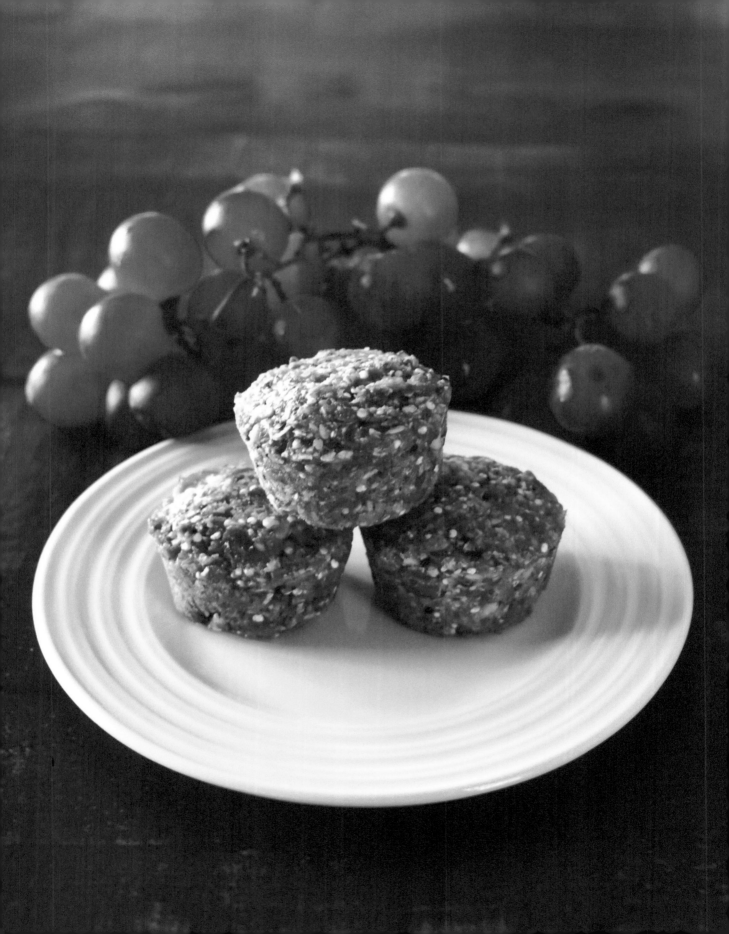

Yogurt

This is a great way to make food for the "good" organisms in your microbiome. Yogurt with probiotics are often recommended when antibiotics disrupt your intestinal system. Making your own yogurt is much easier than one would think and certainly much healthier. It takes time to ferment, but prep time is minimal. For fermentation, a temperature between 85-115°F is required. You can achieve this in a variety of ways by creating a fermentation warming place. You can set your oven on low or warm with the door open (test this first as oven temps vary). Some ovens achieve a temperature between 85 and 115°F by simply having the light on. Another option is to use a slow cooker set on warm, making heating adjustments by setting your yogurt jars on top in a baking pan or on a board, using dishtowels to insulate. Instant Pots are quite popular and include a specific setting for yogurt. It is very difficult to get nondairy yogurt to thicken. Flaxseed not only thickens this yogurt, but also provides more nutrients.

INGREDIENTS AND SUPPLIES

Organic nondairy milk
One (1) capsule of fresh probiotic acidophilus vegetable capsules per cup of milk; each with about 40
    billion CFUs (colony forming units)
2-3 teaspoons of crushed flaxseeds per cup of milk
Clean jars with lids

FERMENTING INSTRUCTIONS

* Preheat and test warming set up to ensure temperature range is between 85-115°F. Temperatures over
    115°F will kill the probiotic colony. Slow cooker or oven set up with temperature maintained between
    85-115°F .

* In a saucepan, bring nondairy milk to a simmer, stirring for about 30 seconds, then remove from heat.
    Allow it cool for about 30 minutes until the temperature is between 85 and 115°F. If you don't have
    thermometer, it should be cool enough to touch (warm, not hot).

* Open probiotic capsules, disperse over the milk, add crushed flaxseed, and whisk gently.

* Pour mixture into jars, cover with lids, and place the jars in the prewarmed setup.

* Allow jars to ferment for 10-12 hours, then place them in the refrigerator.

* Enjoy with fresh or dried fruit/berries, granola, nuts, seeds, cinnamon, nutmeg, date paste/syrup, honey,
    maple syrup, with fruit compote, or lemon curd (See recipes).

Lemon Curd for Yogurt

INGREDIENTS AND SUPPLIES

2 lemons, peeled and seeded
1/4 cup water
1/4-1/3 cup honey, maple syrup, or date syrup
1 tablespoon crushed flaxseeds or whole grain flour

INSTRUCTIONS

Blend ingredients to a puree and serve with yogurt.

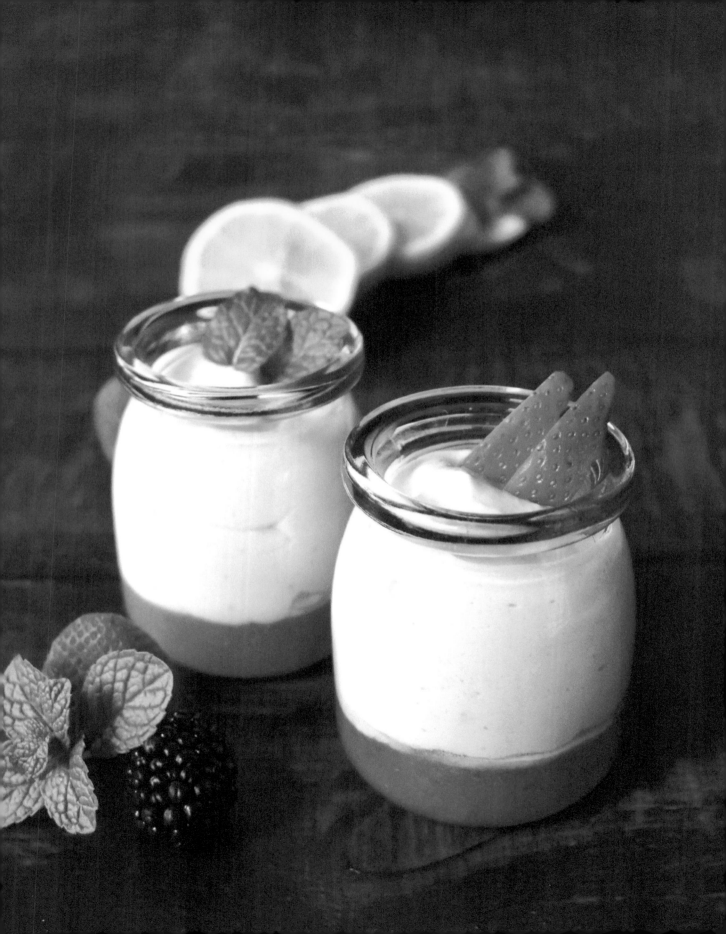

Soups, Stews, Chilies, Curries, Wraps, and Sandwiches

Pumpkin Squash Soup

Daily Dozen Chili

White Bean Potato Soup

Lentil Soup

Hearty Shiitake Barley Soup

Sweet Potato Wraps/Salad

Chickenless Salad Sandwich/Wrap

Tunaless Salad Sandwich/Wrap

Use low sodium vegetable stock, broth, or water in homemade stews, soups, and chilies. Consider making your own vegetable stock (See recipe). Another easy quick broth is made by combining water with miso paste or chickenless bouillon powder (See recipe). Don't hesitate to make soup or stew for dinner. It is one of the most comforting, home-warming meals. Consider serving it with a side salad and garlic bread.

Pumpkin Squash Soup

This is a superhealing, plant-based recreation of Panera's Autumn Squash Soup. It contains a powerful combination of anticancer, anti-inflammatory, antibacterial ingredients that are also used to treat many digestive problems. I make this soup for one of my especially wonderful cancer patients who often craves Panera's squash soup.

BOILING INGREDIENTS

2 cups low sodium vegetable broth, nutritional oil, or water
1/3 cup raw cashews
1 medium butternut squash peeled, seeded, 1/4-to-1/2-inch slices
1 cup mild onion or shallots, sliced or chopped

REMAINING INGREDIENTS

1 cup unsweetened applesauce or 3/4 cup pure apple juice
1 15-ounce can of pure pumpkin
2 tablespoons date sugar, pure honey, or maple syrup
1 teaspoon turmeric
1/2 teaspoon curry powder, optional
1/4 teaspoon ginger
1/2 teaspoon cinnamon
1/2 teaspoon black pepper, ground
A dash or 2 of cayenne pepper, optional

PREPARATION

* In a large pot, add the BOILING INGREDIENTS, then cover to cook/steam until tender for about 20-25 minutes, depending on the thickness of the squash slices. Check with a knife tip to determine doneness.
* Use an immersion blender or transfer ingredients to a blender covered with a lid and towel to purée, then add back to the pot along with the REMAINING INGREDIENTS.
* Bring to a rolling boil. Reduce to simmer for 15-30 minutes.
* Garnish with pumpkin seeds and sprinkle with cinnamon, if desired.
* Serve with green salad and whole grain bread.

Daily Dozen Chili

What I love about this meal is that it includes ingredients from each category of Dr. Michael Greger's Daily Dozen nutritional recommendations. It's a great meal for healing and recovery. This chili is better the next day, and perfect for game days and family gatherings. It may seem like a lot of work, but you can make a large batch to freeze and have on hand for several other meals.

SAUTÉ INGREDIENTS

1 medium onion, chopped
2 bell peppers (green, red, or yellow), chopped
1 cup carrots, chopped
4 cloves garlic, minced or sliced
½ block (4 ounces) tempeh, warmed/steamed and crumbled
1 tablespoon fennel, semicrushed
2 teaspoons basil
2 teaspoons oregano
2-4 tablespoon low sodium soy sauce or dark miso slurry

OTHER INGREDIENTS

2 tablespoons flaxseeds, crushed
1 cup kale, collards and/or turnip greens, chopped
1 cup corn
2 cups black beans or kidney beans, rinsed
2 cups garbanzo beans, rinsed
4-5 cups low sodium vegetable stock or water
2 tablespoons chili powder
1 tablespoon ground cumin
1 teaspoon ground cinnamon
1 tablespoon smoked paprika
1/4 cup raisins, chopped
1-2 tablespoons date paste or date sugar, optional

2 teaspoons ground coriander
1 (8 ounce) can tomato paste
2-3 cups diced tomatoes, with juice
1 teaspoon black pepper, freshly ground

GARNISH OPTIONS

Pumpkin seeds, hempseeds, chopped cilantro, avocado slices, onions, jalapeños, greens, green onions, nondairy cheddar cheese, or sour cream (See easy recipe)

PREPARATION

* Add SAUTÉ INGREDIENTS to a large pot over medium heat, and sauté until onions and peppers are lightly browned, adding liquid as needed.

* Add OTHER INGREDIENTS, except for miso, cover, bring to a short boil, reduce to simmer, stirring occasionally for 2 to 3 hours. Longer cooking time results in thicker chili and richer flavor.

* During last hour of cooking time, set up a buffet of self-serve GARNISH bowls.

* Serve with whole grain garlic bread or corn muffins and a side salad.

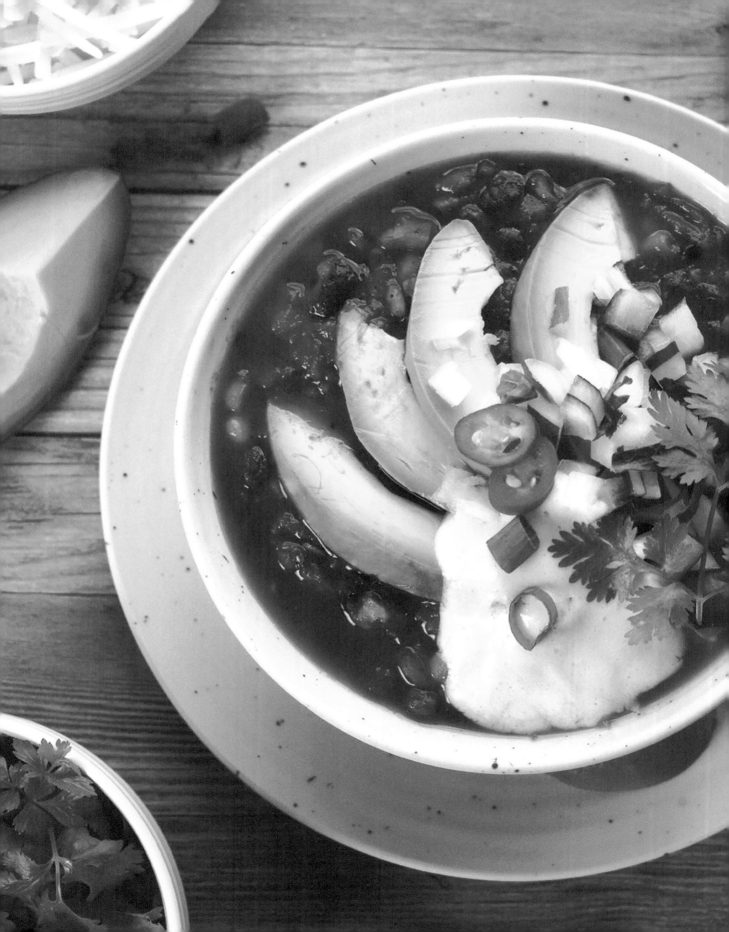

White Bean Corn Potato Stew

This is another hearty healthy meal for a family or social gathering.

SAUTÉ INGREDIENTS

1/2 cup onion, diced
3-4 cloves garlic, minced
1 medium carrot, sliced 1/4 inch
1 celery stalk, sliced/diced, optional

OTHER INGREDIENTS

2 1/2 cups low sodium vegetable stock, broth, or water
1 cup lowfat coconut milk or 1/2 cup cashews simmered in 1/2 cup water, cooled, and
    blended to a cream
3 medium potatoes, peeled and cubed
1 bay leaf

REMAINING INGREDIENTS

2 cups cannellini beans, chickpeas, or navy beans
1 1/2 cups sweet corn or peas
1-2 pinches of cayenne or
    fresh serrano or jalapeño, thinly sliced
2 tablespoons light miso paste slurry (mixed with some warm soup juice)
    Pepper to taste

GARNISH AND SIDES

Fresh chopped parsley, cilantro, green onions, pumpkin seeds, or rosemary.

Serve with side salad or whole grain bread.

PREPARATION

* Add SAUTÉ INGREDIENTS to a pot over medium heat and cook for about 5 minutes to soften and lightly
  brown. Use low sodium vegetable broth or water to keep moist, if needed.
* Then add OTHER INGREDIENTS, bring to a boil, reduce heat, and simmer for 15 minutes. If using
  cashews, simmer 1/2 cup cashews in 1/2 cup of water for 5 minutes, do not drain, cover with a lid, turn
  off heat, soak for 25 minutes, then blend to a cream and add to the pot.
* Add REMAINING INGREDIENTS except for miso to the pot and bring to a simmer for 5-7 minutes.
* Remove from heat and add miso slurry.

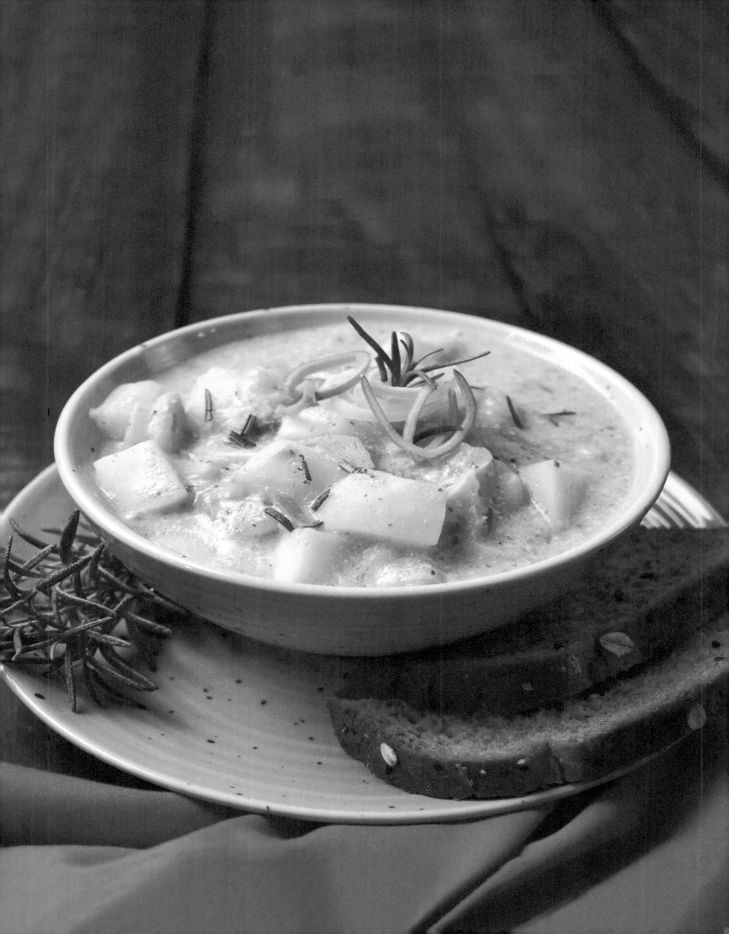

Lentil Soup

Another powerful healing soup full of disease fighting ingredients.

INGREDIENTS

1-2 cups mild onion, chopped
1-2 cups carrots, sliced into 1/4 inch pieces
3-4 garlic cloves, sliced or minced
2 teaspoons ground cumin
1 teaspoon curry powder
1-2 tablespoons of ginger, minced
2 cups diced tomatoes with juice
3/4 cup green or brown lentils, rinsed
1 cup edamame/soybeans or other beans, frozen or fresh
5 cups low sodium vegetable stock, broth, or water
1-2 tablespoons miso paste slurry or low sodium soy sauce
1/4 teaspoon red pepper flakes, optional
1/2 teaspoon fresh ground black pepper, to taste
1-2 cups fresh collards, beet greens or kale, stems removed and chopped

INSTRUCTIONS

* In a large nonstick pot over medium heat, add onions, carrots, and garlic, and cook until the onion is lightly browned. Add broth or water as needed for moisture.

* Add all remaining ingredients, except the greens, cover and return to a boil, reduce heat to simmer, stirring occasionally for 1 hour, then add the greens and heat through for another few minutes.

* Serve with whole grain bread.

Hearty Shiitake Barley Soup

This heart healthy soup is great for a relaxing and enjoying on special days with family.

INGREDIENTS

1-2 boxes low sodium vegetable broth, nutritional oil, or water
1/2 cup barley
1 cup carrots, sliced into 1/4 inch coins
1 cup green beans, peas, or snap peas cut in bite-sized pieces
1 cup celery, sliced in 1/4-inch pieces
2 garlic cloves, minced, or 3/4 teaspoon garlic powder
2 leeks, white and light green parts, 1/4 to 1/2-inch slices
1 turnip, peeled and sliced or chopped
3 medium-sized potatoes, cut into 3/4-inch cubes
   1 1/2 cups shredded cabbage
2 bay leaves
1/2 cup any shiitake or portobello mushrooms, chopped or sliced,
or 1 tablespoon mushroom powder
   1/4 cup fresh parsley, finely chopped
   1 teaspoon dried thyme
1/4 to 1/2 teaspoon pepper
   2 teaspoons lemon juice
2 tablespoons dark miso paste slurry or low sodium soy sauce, to taste/health

PREPARATION

* In a large pot over medium-high heat, add all ingredients as listed, except for miso. Bring to short boil, reduce to simmer, stir occasionally, cooking until vegetables are tender for about 30-40 minutes. Remove from heat, cool for 10 minutes, and add miso.

* Consider serving with whole grain bread and side salad.

Sweet Potato Wraps

INGREDIENTS

8 organic whole grain tortillas
Dark leafy greens such as spinach or watercress
2 cups sweet potatoes, cut into strips or wedges
1 cup onion, sliced

OTHER INGREDIENTS

1 cup lentils, rinsed
1/2 teaspoon cinnamon
1 teaspoon cardamom, ground
1/3 cup chives or green onions, sliced
1/4 teaspoon freshly ground black pepper
1 tablespoon dark miso paste slurry or low sodium soy sauce
1/2 cup pistachios, roughly chopped (can use as a garnish or mix them in)
1/2 cup pomegranate seed berries or raisins (can use as a garnish or mix them in)

MAPLE DRESSING

1/4 cup maple syrup
3 tablespoons cider vinegar
3/4 cup nutritional oil (See recipe)
2 teaspoons miso paste
1/2 teaspoon cinnamon
1 teaspoon Dijon mustard
1 1/2 tablespoons flaxseed, crushed (let set for 10 minutes for thickening)

INSTRUCTIONS

* Preheat oven to 400°F and prepare a parchment lined baking sheet or nonstick baking mat.

* Lay out sweet potatoes and onions on the baking sheet or mat and roast for 20-25 minutes until soft. Check potatoes with a knife tip (can also use an air fryer).

* In a saucepan over medium heat, simmer lentils for 30-35 minutes in water, remove from heat, and drain.

* Combine lentils with remaining OTHER INGREDIENTS in a large bowl.

* Combine MAPLE DRESSING in a small bowl.

* Place a layer of greens then some sweet potato and onion in the center of the tortilla, then add some lentil mixture and drizzle with some of the dressing (or serve lentils mixture on top of a leafy greens salad).

Chickenless Salad Sandwich/Wrap

BASE INGREDIENTS

2 cups of tempeh, 1/2-inch cubes or chickpeas, rinsed, drained, and chopped (other options
  include hearts of palm or jackfruit boiled, drained, and pressed)
1/2 cup celery, thinly sliced or chopped
1/4 cup onion, chopped
3-4 tablespoons raisins
1/4 cup apples, chopped into small cubes/pieces
2 tablespoons walnut or almonds, chopped
1/4 teaspoon curry powder, optional
2 tablespoons fresh parsley or 1/4 teaspoon dried parsley or dill

DRESSING INGREDIENTS

1/2 cup plant-based mayonnaise
2 tablespoons apple cider vinegar
2 tablespoons date syrup or maple syrup
1/4 cup nutritional yeast
2 tablespoons light miso paste or
  2 tablespoons vegetable bouillon (See recipe)
1/2 teaspoon fresh ground pepper

PREPARATION

* Combine BASE INGREDIENTS in a medium sized bowl.

* Combine DRESSING INGREDIENTS in a small bowl, mix well, and add desired amount of
  dressing.

* Create a sandwich or wrap or serve on a bed of lettuce and top with tomato, avocado,
  green onions, walnuts, black pepper, red pepper flakes, alfalfa, or sprouts.

Tunaless Salad Sandwich or Wrap

Good way to incorporate some healthy seaweed with iodine and omega oils.

INGREDIENTS

1/4 cup red onion, finely chopped (consider using a food processor or chopper)
2 cups or 1 can chickpeas, rinsed and roughly chopped, tempeh, steamed/crumbled, or
1/4 cup dill pickle, chopped
2 stalks celery with leaves, finely chopped
1/4 teaspoon celery seeds
1 tablespoon seaweed/nori, crushed, or 1/4 teaspoon kelp powder
2 teaspoons ground or Dijon mustard
2 tablespoons lemon juice
1/2 teaspoon garlic powder
1/4 teaspoon black pepper
1/3-1/2 cup plant-based mayonnaise
1/2 teaspoon Old Bay seasoning, optional

PREPARATION

* Place onion in food processor to partially chop, then add all other ingredients and pulse chop to desired consistency. Do not overdo it, turning it into mush.

* Serve on whole grain bread or wraps and garnish with lettuce leaves, tomato, avocado, onion slices, or sprouts. Can also serve a scoop of this on a salad.

Dinner Selections

Burgers and Grillers

Lentil Tempeh Taco Wraps

Barbecued Vegetables, Grains, and Greens

Plant-Based Meatloaf or Meatballs

Meatloaf Sauce

Stir Fried Vegetables

Portobello Enchiladas

Thai Red Curry

Crabless Crabcake Patties

Orange Salsa Marmalade

King Oyster Mushroom Scallops

Crabless Sushi Rolls

Fishless Taco

Mashed Potatoes

Gravy

Mushroom Bourguignonne

Tempeh, Tofu, or Bean

Stir Fry Meals

Stir Fry Sauces

Sweet BBQ Sauce

Grillable Plant-Based Burgers

It is very difficult, if not impossible to match the flavor of factory-made burgers without the use of chemical additives and high amounts of salt. See if you can make this even better for your taste buds.

INGREDIENTS

1 cup short grain brown rice, cooked as
   recommended (short grain is sticky)
1/2 cup fine cut bulgur or lentils
8 cups water
1 3/4 cups rolled oats
1 1/2 teaspoons xanthan powder, mixed with oats
   (adds sturdiness)

OTHER INGREDIENTS

1 cup onion, chopped
3/4 cup mushrooms (shiitake or portobello) or
   zucchini, chopped
1/2 teaspoon onion powder
1/2 teaspoon garlic powder
1/2 cup sundried tomatoes (If dry, rinse to
   soften) or use 3 tablespoons tomato paste

1 small piece of cooked beet, about 1 inch square,
   chopped (for great color), optional
2 cups or 15-ounces black beans, rinsed and
   roughly chopped
1/2 cup walnuts, finely chopped or hemp seeds
1 teaspoon smoked paprika or plain paprika and
   1/2 teaspoon liquid smoke
1 teaspoon ground black pepper
2 tablespoons dark miso paste slurry or
   2 tablespoons low sodium soy sauce
2 tablespoons balsamic vinegar
3 tablespoons flaxseed, crushed (stickiness)
1/4 cup nutritional yeast
2 tablespoons date sugar or date paste
1/4 cup parsley, basil, or cilantro, fresh and finely
   chopped

PREPARATION

* Preheat oven to 375°F.

* Add rice, bulgur/lentils, and 6 cups of water to a pot, bring to a boil, cover with a lid, reduce heat to simmer for 35 minutes, drain well, cover with a lid, and set aside.

* Add oats and xanthan or guar gum powder to a dry food processor or blender and roughly chop.Transfer to a small bowl.

* To the food processor, add OTHER INGREDIENTS in batches, chop, then transfer to a large mixing bowl.

* Roughly chop rice, bulgur, or lentils and transfer to the mixing bowl.

* Add oat blend and mix well with hands. Wait 5-10 minutes for the flaxseed and xanthan to firm up, then form burger patties and place them on parchment paper or a nonstick baking mat (not foil).

* Bake in the oven for 20 minutes, then transfer to a skillet or grill to lightly brown for one minute on each side (You may need grill spray tp prevent sticking. Resist the urge to overcook on the grill).

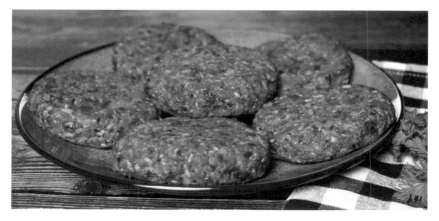

Design Your Own Plant-Based Burger

There are so many ways to make a plant-based burger. The base can be made from any combination of bulgur wheat, black beans, chickpeas, lentils, tempeh, brown rice, quinoa, oats, tofu, eggplant, zucchini, or even sweet or white potato. For color, use sundried tomatoes, red beets, beet powder, beet juice, or tomato paste. To add some healthy wholesome oils, add avocado, ground flax, walnuts, or seed butters. For a beefy flavor, add mushrooms. Go easy on the liquid ingredients like soy sauce, balsamic vinegar, and plant-based or vegan Worcestershire sauce as they can make a burger mushy. Add any spices or greens you want like parsley, basil, dill, thyme, or cilantro. Be creative with your toppings. Add the classic dill or sweet pickles, lettuce, tomato, ketchup, and mustard. Other toppings can include caramelized onions, tempeh bacon, sautéed mushrooms, nondairy mayonnaise, cucumbers, pickled red onions, sprouts, or avocado. Also try sauces like honey mustard, cilantro-lime, BBQ, nondairy ranch dressing and thousand island, or even horseradish sauce. Serve with a salad, baked or air fried fries, potato salad, coleslaw, yellow rice and beans, or homemade baked beans.

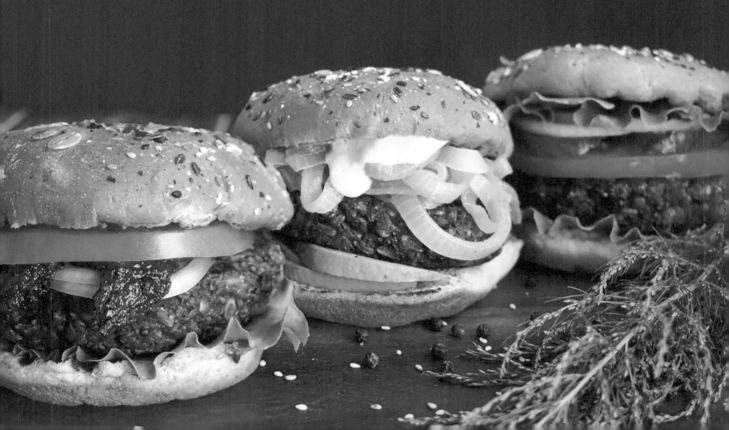

Tempeh or Lentil Taco Wraps

You can easily make tacos from any of the vegetables you have in your refrigerator or garden. Just have tortillas on hand. This is one of my go-to recipes that makes the family happy and when we are short on time for planning dinner.

INGREDIENTS
4-5 organic whole grain tortillas

SAUTÉ INGREDIENTS

1 ½ cups red onion, sliced
3 cloves garlic or 1/4 teaspoon garlic powder
1 bell pepper, any color, sliced
1 cup tempeh, steamed and crumbled or
    cooked lentils
1 cup black beans, chickpeas, or pinto beans
1 cup corn, frozen or fresh
1 teaspoon ground cumin
2 teaspoons chili powder
1/2 teaspoon paprika
1/2 teaspoon oregano
1 tablespoon low sodium soy sauce
1 tablespoon lime juice
1/2 teaspoon fresh ground black pepper
    or 1-2 pinches of cayenne pepper, optional

1/2 cup low sodium vegetable broth, nutritional
    oil (See recipe), or water

UNFRIED BEANS, OPTIONAL

1-2 cups black beans, chickpeas or pinto beans, rinsed and blended in a food processor with a little water, lime juice, miso paste, salsa, tomato, green chilies, jalapeño peppers, or pepper flakes, to taste. Have fun with it.

GARNISH AND SIDE DISHES—Self-Serve Buffet Style

2 avocados, sliced, or guacamole
1 cup cherry tomatoes, sliced
1 cup cilantro, chopped, or parsley, fresh
4-6 lime wedges
1 cup plant-based sour cream (Recipe available)
Salsa or hot chili sauce

PREPARATION

* In a large skillet over medium heat, sauté onion, garlic, and bell pepper,

* Add remaining SAUTÉ INGREDIENTS and simmer for 20-30 minutes, adding broth as needed for moisture.

* For UNFRIED BEANS, add beans and desired ingredients to a food processor to blend to desired consistency.

* Lay out tortillas and prepare garnishes and side dishes for self-serve buffet. Done!

Barbecued Vegetables, Grains, and Greens

Inspired by PlantPure Nation and Kim Campbell at plantpurenation.com where you will find many other excellent WFPB educational resources and recipe ideas. This barbecue sauce recipe is very tasty with grains, coleslaw, salad, rice, hash browns, or in a wrap and is very quick to prepare.

INGREDIENTS

1 cup quinoa, whole grain-brown rice, barley, or farro

SAUCE INGREDIENTS

3-4 cloves garlic, minced or ¼ teaspoon dry garlic powder

1/2 cup organic ketchup (no high fructose corn syrup)

1 tablespoon dry mustard

1 tablespoon chili powder

1 ½ teaspoons smoked paprika

1 teaspoon liquid smoke

1/4 cup low sodium soy sauce

3 tablespoons date sugar or date syrup

1/3 cup umami sauce or plant-based Worcestershire sauce (no anchovies)

VEGETABLES

1 cup bell pepper, chopped

1/2 cup onions, chopped

2 cups or 1 can black beans

2 cups corn, fresh or frozen

1 jalapeño, serrano, or other spicy pepper, optional

PREPARATION

* Prepare grains as recommended. If using rice, add 1 cup per 6 cups of water to a pot, bring to a boil, cover with a lid, reduce heat to simmer for 35 minutes, drain well to remove potential toxins, and set aside on warm burner to steam and fluff.

* Prepare ranch dressing for salad, optional (See recipe).

* Combine SAUCE INGREDIENTS in a saucepan over medium heat, stir, and bring to a simmer for 10-15 minutes.

* Add VEGETABLES to the saucepan with the sauce and simmer for another 10-15 minutes until thickened.

* Pour barbecued vegetables over grains or greens or alongside them and garnish with avocado, green onions, or sprouts.

Plant-Based Meatloaf or Meatballs

This is a great home-cooked meal. Consider serving with mashed potatoes and carrots, green beans, peas, asparagus, Brussels sprouts, or broccoli and a salad.

GENERAL INGREDIENTS

1/3 cup short grain brown rice and/or bulgur, rinsed and cooked per recommendation.
4 cups water
2 tablespoons crushed flaxseeds in 3 (not 6) tablespoons water, let set for at least 10 minutes to thicken
1 1/2 cups oats
1 teaspoon xanthan gum

OTHER INGREDIENTS – consider using a food processor for chopping and mixing to save time

1/2 cup walnuts, 1/2 avocado, or 1/3 cup pumpkin seeds finely chopped
1 cup of tempeh, steamed and crumbled or chopped
1 cup black beans, rinsed and chopped
2 cups mushrooms, chopped
1 cup onion, chopped
3 cloves garlic, minced or thinly sliced
2 tablespoons low sodium soy sauce or dark miso paste
1 tablespoon balsamic vinegar
1/2 teaspoon salt, optional (soybean tempeh above may help buffer salt damaging effects)
2 tablespoon Italian seasoning (See recipe)
2 teaspoons fennel, semicrushed, mortar and pestle or coffee bean grinder work well
2 tablespoons nutritional yeast, optional
1/4 cup fresh parsley, finely chopped, optional
1/4 cup whole grain bread crumbs or 1 cup whole grain piece of bread torn into small pieces
1 teaspoon fresh ground pepper

PREPARATION

* Preheat oven to 400°F. Prepare a nonstick baking mat, parchment-lined baking sheet, or a nonstick loaf pan.

* In a pot or saucepan, combine rice and/or bulgur and 4-5 cups of water, cover with a lid, bring to a boil, reduce to a simmer for 35 minutes, drain well, cover with lid and set aside.

* Combine flaxseeds and water in a small cup or bowl for 5-10 minutes until gelled.

* Place oats and xanthan in a dry blender, blend to a rough flour, and set aside.

* Add walnuts, avocado, or pumpkin seeds to a food processor and chop/blend.

* Warm tempeh by steaming it or placing it in the microwave for 15 seconds, then break up into pieces and transfer to the food processor.

* Add remaining OTHER INGREDIENTS to the food processor in batches and pulse-chop to a rough texture resembling ground meat, transfer to a large mixing bowl along with flax gel, oat flour mix, rice and/or bulgur, and use hands to mix well.

* *For meatloaf*, form into 2 or 3 loaves. Smaller loaves bake faster. Spread Meatloaf Sauce Recipe or BBQ sauce over the "meat" loaves. For 2 loaves, bake for about 50 minutes. For 3 loaves, bake for about 35 minutes.

* *For meatballs,* skip the sauce and roll mix into balls. Meatball baking time will vary from about 15 minutes to 40 minutes, depending on size. Watch for light browning and firmness.

Meatloaf Sauce

MEATLOAF SAUCE INGREDIENTS , optional (this is a great sauce, but you can use any BBQ sauce)
1 ½ cups organic ketchup (recipe available)
1 cup date sugar or ¾ cup date paste or maple syrup
2 teaspoons vegan Worcestershire sauce (no anchovies).

PREPARATION
Combine MEATLOAF SAUCE INGREDIENTS in a small saucepan over medium heat, bring to a simmer for 2 minutes, then remove from heat.

Stir Fried Vegetables

RICE
1 cup brown rice or brown rice noodles or any
  whole grains

TEMPEH, FIRM TOFU, OR SOYBEANS (any legumes)
1/2-1 block tempeh or tofu, thawed, pressed, and
  cut into bite-size pieces or crumbled

SAUCE
1/4 cup rice wine vinegar
1/4 cup low sodium soy sauce
1/4 cup low sodium vegetable stock, broth, or
  water
2 teaspoons nutritional yeast
3 cloves garlic, minced
2 tablespoons fresh ginger, minced

2 teaspoons tahini
3 tablespoons date syrup or maple syrup
1 tablespoon flour for thickening
1 teaspoon hot chili sauce, optional

STIR-FRY VEGETABLES
1 large carrot, shredded
1 cup sweet onion
3 cups broccoli cut up in bite-size pieces
1/2 red bell pepper
1 cup mushrooms, bok choy, snow pea pods, bean
  sprouts, zucchini, or cabbage

GARNISH
1/2 cup green onion, sliced diagonally
¼ cup cilantro or parsley, chopped
1 teaspoon sesame seeds

PREPARATION
* In a saucepan, combine rice and 6 cups of water, and cook for 35 minutes, drain well, cover with a lid, and set aside to steam 10 minutes more.
* Place tempeh in a medium-large nonstick pot over medium heat and cook until lightly browned.
* Combine SAUCE INGREDIENTS in a medium saucepan over medium heat, bring to a short boil, then remove from heat.
* Add STIR-FRY VEGETABLES to the pot with the tempeh or tofu, add low sodium vegetable broth, stock, or water and vegetables in order listed, cover and allow to steam a minute or two, then stir and toss for a couple minutes more and remove from heat.
* On individual plates, layer the rice/noodles, stir-fry vegetables, and garnish with sesame seeds, sliced green onion, cilantro, or parsley.

Portobello Enchiladas

This recipe is a huge hit with plenty of flavor, color, and pure wow! Choose from any of the sauces or toppings that follow this recipe. We enjoy the Enchilada Red Sauce (though spicy), the Verde Sauce, and a drizzle of the nondairy Queso Cheese Sauce. You can prepare your sauces, bean spread, and sliced vegetables early in the day or the day before, then assemble your meal 30 minutes before serving guests.

GENERAL INGREDIENTS

4-6 whole grain tortillas

1 cup whole grain rice (or other whole grain), cook rice as recommended below

3 cups low sodium vegetable stock, broth, or water

FILLER INGREDIENTS

1 cup onion, sliced

3 cloves garlic, sliced or minced

4 cups portobello mushrooms, sliced strips

1 cup cabbage, zucchini, eggplant, or cauliflower, thinly sliced strips

1 cup corn, fresh or frozen

1 teaspoon chili powder

1 teaspoon cumin

1 tablespoon lime juice

BEAN PASTE INGREDIENTS

1/4 cup salsa, pico, or enchilada red sauce (recipe available)

1½-2 cups black beans, rinsed and blended or mashed

2 teaspoons lime juice

GARNISH AND SIDES OPTIONS

Enchilada red sauce or your favorite salsa/pico, Verde Sauce, nondairy Queso Cheese Sauce (See recipe), chopped cilantro, sliced avocados, diced fresh tomatoes, chopped onions, lettuce/greens, nondairy cheddar and Jack cheeses, or nondairy sour cream (See recipe).

PREPARATION

* Preheat oven to 375°F

* In a saucepan over medium heat, add rice and 6 cups of water, bring to a boil, reduce to simmer for 35 minutes, drain well, cover with a lid, and set aside on warm burner for about 15 minutes to steam and fluff.

* Place FILLER INGREDIENTS in a large nonstick skillet over medium heat, cook for 5-7 minutes, adding small amount of stock, broth, or water, as needed until lightly browned/softened.

* Spread a thin layer of salsa, Enchilada Red Sauce, or pico, over the bottom of a casserole dish.

* Add ¼ cup of salsa or Enchilada Red Sauce to the food processor along with the BEAN PASTE INGREDIENTS and blend to a spread.

* Take each tortilla and spread it with some bean paste, then add some FILLER INGREDIENTS to the middle 1/3 and roll up each tortilla and place it in the casserole dish seam side down.

* Pour some verde sauce, red sauce, or queso sauce over enchiladas, scatter some nondairy cheese on top and bake for 10-15 minutes until the cheese melts a little.

* Prepare each plate with a side serving of rice.

* Serve with or over some greens, and garnish with your choice of avocado, diced tomatoes, hot peppers, hot sauce, nondairy sour cream, or cilantro.

Thai Red Curry

A nice dish for incorporating some sea vegetables and many other great disease-fighting nutrients.

BASE INGREDIENTS

1-2 cups firm tofu, thawed and pressed, or tempeh, sliced or cubed
2 cups brown rice (or other whole grain), rinsed and cooked as recommended below

CURRY VEGETABLES

2 carrots, sliced
1 cup onion, ¼ inch wedges
2 tablespoons fresh ginger, grated or minced
4 cloves garlic, minced, pressed, or thinly sliced
1 red, yellow, or orange bell pepper, ¼ inch slices
1 cup broccoli, cut in bite-sized pieces
3-4 cups bok choy, kale, or spinach, cut into bite-sized pieces

CURRY SAUCE INGREDIENTS

2-3 cups low fat coconut milk
1 cup nondairy milk
3-4 tablespoons Thai red curry paste (See recipe for homemade Red Curry Paste)
4 lemongrass sticks/cores, peeled and twisted to release flavor or 5 kaffir lime leaves
½ lime or lemon blended, optional
¼ cup low sodium soy sauce, to taste/health
2-3 tablespoons date sugar, date syrup, or maple syrup, adjust to taste/health
½ sheet or 2 tablespoons seaweed—nori or dulce—torn into pieces or chopped
2-3 tablespoons whole grain flour, sprinkled over sauce to thicken

GARNISH OPTIONS:

Thai basil leaves or cilantro, chopped. Lime or lemon wedges, fresh jalapeños, serrano's, or red pepper flakes

PREPARATION

* For 2 cups rice, add 12 cups of water, bring to a boil, cover with a lid, reduce heat to simmer for 35 minutes, drain well to remove potential toxins, then set aside on warm burner (heat turned off).
* Prepare Red Curry Paste, if needed.
* While rice is cooking, prepare the CURRY VEGETABLES and set aside.
* In a large nonstick pot over medium heat, lightly brown tofu or tempeh, then add chunky vegetables, except for leafy greens (bok choy, kale, spinach) and cook for 5-8 minutes.
* Add CURRY SAUCE INGREDIENTS to the pot, bring to a simmer for a few minutes until thickened, then remove from heat and add leafy greens.
* Pour vegetable curry over rice, and top with desired garnishes.

Crabless Crabcakes

Seafood flavor achieved with seaweed providing plenty of iodine and many other healthy healing ingredients. Serve alongside some roasted vegetables, a side salad, or soup. Try some *Orange Salsa Marmalade* on your crabcake (See recipe).

BASE INGREDIENTS
1 cup chickpeas, chopped
1 cup hearts of palm, rinsed, drained, cut into
    1/2 inch pieces
2 teaspoons Old Bay seasoning
4 garlic cloves, minced or 1 1/4 teaspoons
    garlic powder
1 tablespoon nutritional yeast
1 teaspoon smoked paprika
1/2 teaspoon pepper, fresh ground

*SAUTÉ INGREDIENTS – easy to use food
processor to chop into small pieces*
1/4 cup mild onion, chopped
1 stalk of celery, chopped
1/2 bell pepper, chopped

1/2 cup corn, chopped
2 tablespoons quinoa
1/4 cup seaweed, torn or crushed (small pieces)

OTHER INGREDIENTS
2 tablespoons light miso paste slurry or 1/2
    teaspoon natural salt with soy powder, soybeans,
    or tempeh
2 tablespoons flaxseed, crushed
4 tablespoons warm water
3/4 cup whole grain panko, breadcrumbs, or bread,
    torn into small pieces
2 tablespoons cornmeal or hemp seeds
1 teaspoon xanthan powder for added firmness,
    optional

GARNISH
Lemon wedges, sliced green onion, chives, or parsley

PREPARATION

* Preheat oven to 400°F and prepare a large parchment lined baking sheet or a baking mat.

* Prepare Orange Salsa Marmalade (See recipe).

* Add BASE INGREDIENTS to a food processor, chop into small pieces, and transfer to a large mixing bowl.

* Add SAUTÉ INGREDIENTS to the food processor, chop into small pieces, and transfer to a skillet to cook until softened, then transfer to the mixing bowl.

* In a small bowl, combine miso paste, flaxseed, and warm water. Mix to combine, allow to set for 10 minutes to gel, then add to mixing bowl.

* Add OTHER INGREDIENTS to the mixing bowl and combine well by hand.

* Form into crab cake patties 2-3 inches wide by 1/2 inch thick, or form into 1 inch bite-sized, semiflattened appetizer balls, and place on a baking mat or parchment lined baking sheet.

* Bake crab cake patties for 15-20 minutes. Bake bite-sized balls for 8-10 minutes, until lightly browned. Consider encrusting them by transferring to a large nonstick skillet with a spritz of oil and braise for about a minute on each side.

* Top with orange salsa marmalade.

Orange Salsa Marmalade

Unforgettable topping for crabcakes. Can also be enjoyed as a spread, jam, or a dip.

INGREDIENTS

2 small or 1 large orange
1/4 cup onion, chopped
1/4 cup bell pepper, chopped
1 teaspoon lemon juice
1-2 jalapeño or serrano peppers, finely chopped, optional, but delicious
1/2-2/3 cup honey
1/4 teaspoon xanthan or 1/2 teaspoon agar

PREPARATION

* For thin skinned oranges, slice off about half of the skin, slice into 1/2 inch sections to remove large seeds, and transfer to a food processor. For thick skinned spongy oranges, use an apple peeler or grater to peel and retain half of the outer skin layer. Peel away some thick spongy underlayer and discard. Slice orange into 1/2 inch sections to remove large seeds and transfer skin and orange to a food processor. Chop into small pieces.

* Add remaining ingredients, except for honey to the food processor, chop to desired consistency, transfer to a saucepan over medium heat, add honey, and bring to a simmer for about 5 minutes.

* To thicken, add xanthan powder, optional depending on juiciness of oranges (5 minutes to thicken).

King Oyster Scallops

It is shocking how much these mushrooms can actually taste like scallops. Even my 5th generation commercial fisherman husband from Maine will admit this. We enjoy them seared and served on top of the Creamy Cauliflower Pasta. Oyster mushrooms contain nearly 3% lovastatin which may actually lower your cholesterol levels by nearly 30%.

MARINADE INGREDIENTS

2-3 large king oyster mushrooms, stems sliced 1 inch thick (found at Wegman's)
2 cups warm vegetable broth
1/4 cup soy sauce
1/4 cup or 1 sheet of seaweed, torn or crumbled (nori or dulse)

LEMON MISO SAUCE

2 garlic cloves, minced or ¼ teaspoon garlic powder
1 tablespoons miso paste slurry (mixed with 1 tablespoons warm water)
1-2 teaspoons lemon, juiced
2 teaspoons of plant-based butter, optional
Sprinkle with a little seafood seasoning, optional

PREPARATION

* Combine MARINADE INGREDIENTS and allow to soak for at least 2 hours or preferably overnight.

* In a non-stick skillet over medium heat, lightly brown "scallop" edges, using a little broth or a spritzer of oil.

* In a small saucepan, heat LEMON MISO SAUCE, pour over scallops, and heat through.

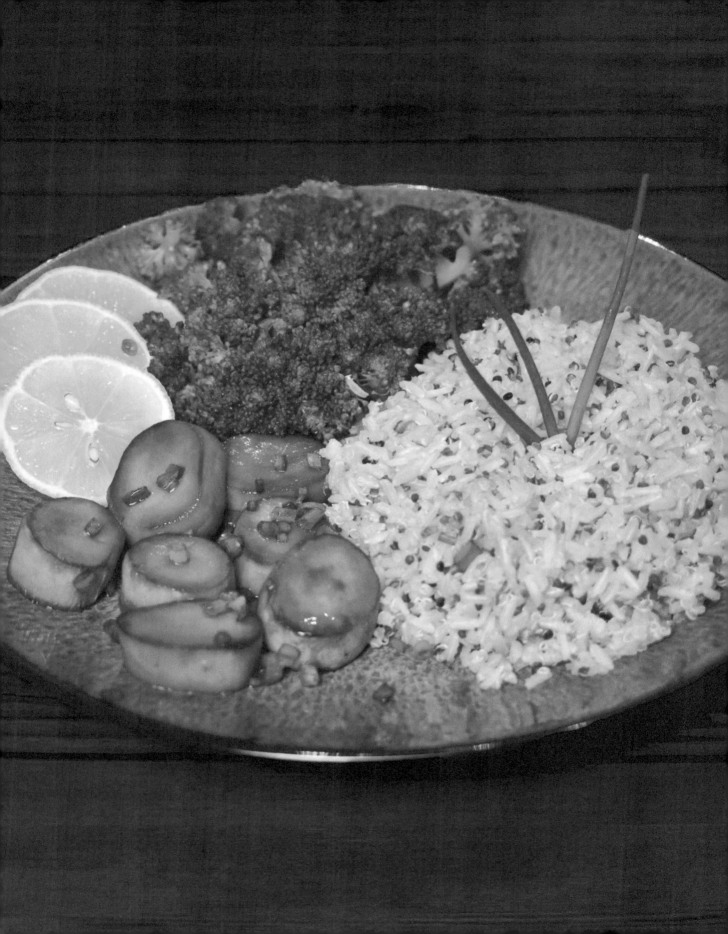

Crabless Sushi Rolls

You can make this as a sushi salad or brave it and make sushi rolls. It's not that hard if you have seen it done or watch a video on how it's done (found online). If this is your first time, be sure you have a bamboo sushi roller. Find it online or in Asian markets. This recipe was inspired by Andrew Olson at OneIngredientChef.com.

SUSHI RICE INGREDIENTS – Can be made ahead and refrigerated

2 cups short grain brown rice
7 cups low sodium vegetable broth or water
3 tablespoons rice vinegar
1 tablespoon pure honey or maple syrup
½ teaspoon salt + 1 tsp soy powder or some soybeans/tempeh

"CRAB" FILLER INGREDIENTS – Can be made ahead and refrigerated

½ cup raw cashews (simmered and soaked) or plant-based mayonnaise
1 block of warm crumbled tempeh, 1 ½ cups chickpeas or hearts of palm, rinsed and pressed to remove water
1 ½ tablespoons lemon juice
2 teaspoons tahini
1 tablespoon chili garlic sauce, or use chili hot sauce and some garlic powder
½ cup cabbage, purple or green, sliced
½ cup carrots, sliced
1 sheet of nori seaweed, torn into pieces
1 tablespoon low sodium soy sauce
¼ teaspoon fresh ground pepper

"SUSHI" ROLLS INGREDIENTS

2-3 sheets of nori seaweed, cut in half for small bite-sized rolls (crab filler—above)
1 cucumber, 8 inches long, thin sliced strips
1 large carrot, 4 inches long, thin sliced strips
1 cup spinach leaves
1 avocado, thinly sliced
1 teaspoon sesame seeds, black or white

GARNISHES

Low sodium soy sauce with some water for dipping, ginger, wasabi, and sliced green onions

PREPARATION

* Add brown rice and 12 cups of water to a saucepan over high heat, cover with a lid, reduce to a simmer, cook for 35 minutes, drain well, cover with a lid, and set on a warm burner for about 15 minutes, then place in the refrigerator to cool.

* When ready to assemble, remove rice from the fridge and add rice vinegar, honey, and miso and mix well.

* In a saucepan, add cashews with 1 cup of water, cover with a lid, bring to a simmer, remove from heat, and allow cashews to soak for 30-minutes. Reserve liquid while straining over a bowl measuring one-half cup of liquid to add to a blender along with the cashews. Blend to a smooth cream.

* In a food processor, combine the SUSHI "CRAB" FILLER INGREDIENTS, except for the cream, gently pulse/chop a few times, then add cashew cream and pulse to a fine chunky mix (not mush).

* For assembling, you will need a bowl of cool water, plastic wrap, and a towel to rinse, wipe, and wet fingers. Also, you will need it to clean and wet the knife blade. Cut nori sheets in half and lay one on a cutting board with the rough side up. Add about 1/4 to 1/2 inch rice under and along nori edge opposite side from you. Overlapping rice will be the glue to seal the rolls.

* For rice on the outside: You will need two areas for assembling. Place plastic wrap on bamboo next to seaweed on cutting board with a thin layer of rice on top. You can first sprinkle some sesame seeds over the plastic if you want them on the outside, then gently flip seaweed with rice from the cutting board over onto the plastic seeded wrap. Add small amount of filler and cucumber along the end closest to you with about 1/2 inch of seaweed uncovered.

* For avocado on the outside: two surfaces as above, but layer seaweed, then rice, then avocado strips, and lay plastic wrap over avocado and gently flip over onto plastic covered bamboo. Then add small amount of filler and cucumber along the end closest to you with about 1/2 inch of seaweed uncovered.

* For seaweed on the outside: This is easier with only one work surface, seaweed on the bamboo with a thin layer of rice on it. Then add small amount of filler and cucumber along the end closest to you with about 1/2 inch of seaweed uncovered.

* As you begin to roll with the bamboo, use a wet knife to press contents inside and against roller to help pack contents in place, remove knife and finish rolling while gently pressing bamboo and pulling plastic wrap out and away until edges of nori come together with overlapping rice acting as glue to seal the roll. Press firmly and push in ends a little while wrapped in bamboo to pack. To slice, cover the roll with cling wrap, hold securely, and slice with a clean, wet, sharp knife blade in a quick slicing motion.

* Use low sodium soy sauce mixed with some wasabi for dipping. Garnish with ginger and more seeds if desired. Consider adding some crunch by adding whole grain panko to a skillet, drizzle with a small amount of veggie butter, briefly sauté, and add it to the top of your sushi.

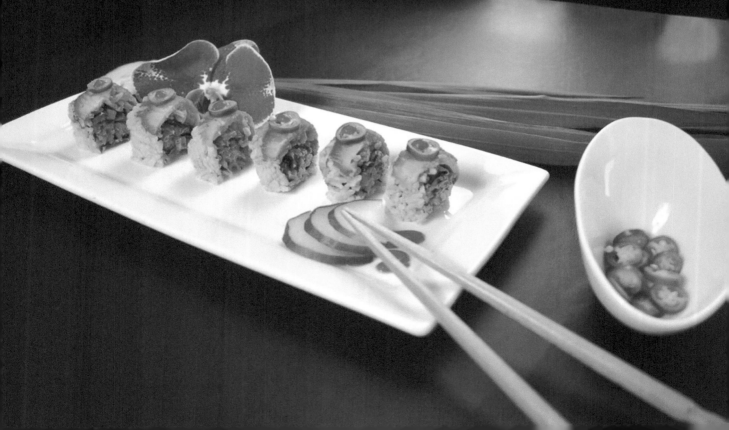

Fishless Tacos

This recipe provides the taste of seafood without the contaminants and includes the great nutrients found in sea vegetables. Consider marinated, seared tofu without batter as an easy alternate to hearts of palm. Serve with a side of whole grains (quinoa mix), cumin lime slaw, or baked fries.

INGREDIENTS

1 can of hearts of palm stalks (found in the canned vegetables aisle or online) or marinated and seared tofu

4-6 organic whole grain or corn tortillas

HEARTS OF PALM MARINADE

1/4 cup ground seaweed-nori sheets, crushed, or 1 ½ teaspoons kelp powder

1 cup water

2 tablespoons low sodium soy sauce

1 teaspoon rice vinegar

1 teaspoon lime juice

1/4 teaspoon garlic powder

1/8 teaspoon ground black pepper

HEARTS OF PALM BATTER INGREDIENTS

1/2 cup whole grain flour or cornmeal

1/2 teaspoon ground cumin

1/2 teaspoon chili powder

1 tablespoon light miso paste slurry

1/8 teaspoon fresh ground pepper

1/2 cup water

CABBAGE SLAW – MAKE AHEAD

2 cups cabbage, thinly shredded

2 tablespoons seaweed-nori, crushed

1/4 cup red onion, thinly sliced

2 cloves garlic, minced

1/4 cup lime juice

2 teaspoons honey

1 teaspoon cumin

1/4 cup cilantro, chopped

1 tablespoon light miso paste slurry, optional

SAUCE INGREDIENTS

1 cup plant-based sour cream or mayonnaise (See recipes)

2 tablespoons adobo sauce with chipotle peppers or other hot sauce

2 tablespoons lime juice

2 teaspoons honey

1 tablespoon light miso paste, soy sauce, or ¼ teaspoon salt + 1 teaspoon soy powder or some soybeans

GARNISH AND SIDES OPTIONS - Self-serve, buffet style works well

Chopped tomatoes or salsa, cilantro, black beans, roasted or grilled corn, lime wedges, jalapeño peppers, or avocado.

PREPARATION

* Combine the HEARTS OF PALM MARINADE, then use the side of a wide knife to semiflatten or cut in half hearts of palm stalk (1 inch pieces). Soak them in marinade for 30 or more minutes. For stronger flavor, cover and refrigerate overnight.

* Preheat oven to 375°F with rack set in upper middle section of oven and prepare a parchment lined baking sheet or nonstick baking mat.

* Combine dry HEARTS OF PALM BATTER INGREDIENTS then add water and adjust, if necessary to achieve a creamy consistency.

* Dip hearts of palm in batter to coat and place them on a baking sheet and bake until lightly browned for 15-20 minutes.

* Add SAUCE INGREDIENTS to a blender and blend to a creamy consistency.

* Assemble tacos by placing battered palm pieces in the center of tortillas with cabbage slaw, dressing, and desired garnishes.

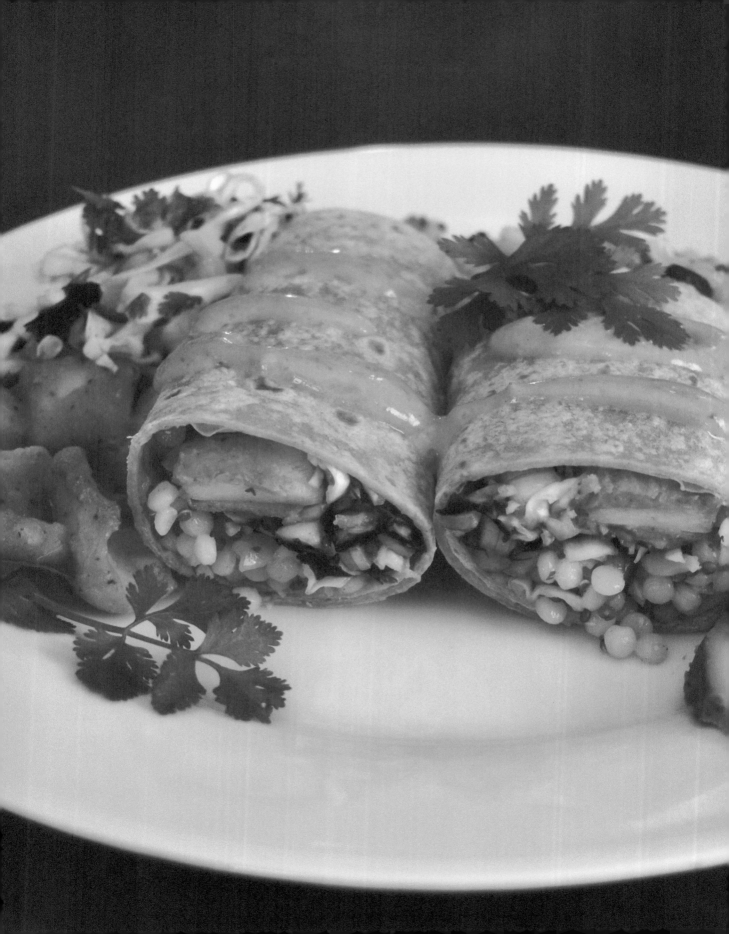

Taking care of people in their homes creates a personal connection where you learn a lot about family members. One of the things many people seem to have in common is their love of "meat" and potatoes (and gravy, see recipe). This section is especially focused on them. Along with the "meat" replacement options listed below, consider adding a side of vegetables like carrots, broccoli, asparagus, peas, roasted vegetables, or even a side salad.

Mashed Potatoes (or Mashed Cauliflower)

Mashed potatoes are one thing many families enjoy, especially over the holidays. They are an excellent source of nutrients as long as you don't add dairy or animal forms of butter, milk, cheese, bacon, or sour cream. All of these can be replaced with plant-based options (See recipes).

INGREDIENTS
4 medium potatoes and or 4-5 cups cauliflower, chopped
1/2 cup low sodium vegetable broth, water, or plain nondairy milk, adjust as needed
1-2 tablespoon white miso paste slurry (mix well with equal parts warm water before adding)
Garnish with: chives, green onions, nondairy cheddar cheese, sour cream, or tempeh or tofu bacon

PREPARATION
* Wash, remove eyes, and partially peel potatoes. Skins provide additional nutritional benefits.
* Slice potatoes into 1/2-inch slices and boil for about 12 minutes in water or vegetable broth.
  Test with knife tip for doneness.
* Drain liquid and return to pot, add miso and milk and mash or blend to desired consistency.
* See gravy recipe.

Gravy

Serve over mashed potatoes and stuffing with steamed vegetables for a delicious home-cooked meal. This gravy can be created to taste like poultry or beef gravy. Using broth or nondairy milk, light miso paste, and cooking onions just until softened results in a lighter colored gravy. Using richer soy (tamari), darker miso paste, vegetable stock, porcini mushroom powder, and caramelizing (browning) onions makes the gravy darker and more beeflike.

BASE INGREDIENTS

1 cup onion, sliced or chopped

3-4 cloves of garlic, minced or sliced

2 cups mushrooms, cremini, portobello, or shiitake, sliced (separately sauté 1 cup mushroom slices, to add back later, if desired)

½ teaspoon fresh ground black pepper

OTHER INGREDIENTS

1 teaspoon fresh rosemary or 1 tablespoon parsley, minced

4 cups low sodium mushroom or vegetable stock, broth, or nondairy milk

1 tablespoon nutritional yeast

2-3 tablespoons whole grain flour sprinkled over gravy, whisk while heating, to thickness preference

2 tablespoons dark miso paste slurry, vegetable chickenlees/beefless bouillon (See recipes), umami, or soy sauce

PREPARATION

* In a large skillet over medium heat, add ½ cup stock or broth and BASE INGREDIENTS, and cook until onions and mushrooms until they are lightly browned. Remove from heat.

* Add 1 cup stock/broth to a blender and add cooked onion mixture, and blend to a purée.

* Return mixture to the skillet, add 3 ½ cups stock or broth, and return to a simmer over medium heat.

* Shake nutritional yeast and flour over the mixture. Stir until bubbly and thickened as desired.

* Remove from heat, and add miso, bouillon, or soy sauce.

Mushroom Bourguignonne over Baked Potato, Mashed Potatoes, or Mashed Cauliflower

Porcini mushrooms are an ultimate beefy flavor mushroom. They are usually sold dried, not fresh. Serve this recipe over potatoes with broccoli, peas, or a salad on the side.

MASHED POTATOES OR CAULIFLOWER

3-4 medium potatoes, 3/4 inch slices or steamed cauliflower

1/2-1 cup low sodium broth or unsweetened, plain nondairy milk

1 tablespoons light miso slurry

INGREDIENTS

2 cups yellow onion, puréed

3 tablespoons dried porcini mushrooms blended to a powder or soaked

1 cup portobello, shiitake, or cremini mushrooms

4 cloves garlic, minced, pressed, or sliced

1 cup portobello, shiitake, or cremini mushrooms, sliced

1 cup carrots, sliced 1/4 inch thick

1/2 cup jackfruit, seeded, simmered, and drainied, to reduce brine, optional for texture

1 bell pepper, chopped

1 celery rib, sliced or 2 pinches of celery seed

4-5 cups mushroom or vegetable broth

1 cup shallots, sliced (or pearl onions)

2 bay leaves

1 teaspoon dried thyme

1 teaspoon dried oregano

1 teaspoon fresh ground pepper

2 tablespoons tomato paste or tomato sauce

1 tablespoon nutritional yeast

2 teaspoon cocoa

1/2 cup organic dry red wine
(there are nonalcoholic wines)

1/3 cup low sodium soy sauce, adjust to taste/health or 2 tablespoons of dark miso paste slurry

2-3 tablespoons whole grain flour for thickening

GARNISH

Chopped fresh chives or parsley for garnish

PREPARATION

* Prepare mashed potatoes or steamed mashed cauliflower, add low sodium broth or milk, and miso, then mash or blend. Cover and set aside to keep warm.

* In a large nonstick skillet or pot over medium heat, add puréed onions and simmer to caramelize for about 20 minutes. No oil is needed if heat is kept at medium low.

* If using dried porcini mushrooms, either blend to a powder or soak in liquid for 30 minutes, then blend with 1 cup of mushrooms to a puree and add to carmamelized onions.

* Add remaining INGREDIENTS, except for flour and simmer for 20 minutes until the carrots are tender. Adjust to desired thickness with flour.

* Serve over baked potato, mashed potatoes, or mashed auliflower and top with some mushroom sauce.

* Garnish with chives or parsley and serve with broccoli, peas, and/or a side salad.

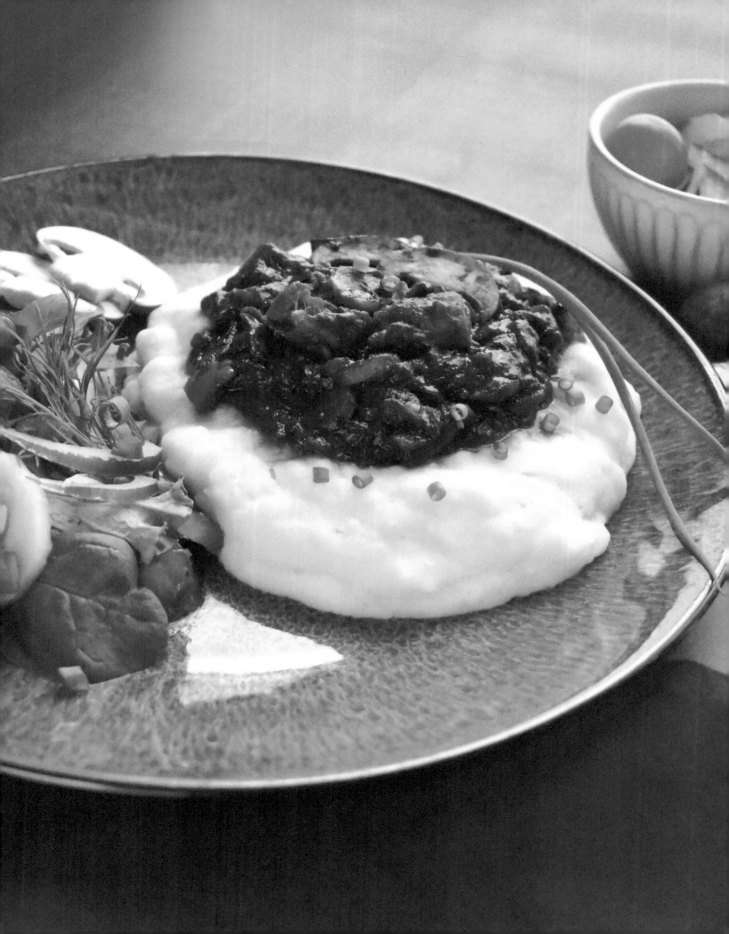

TEMPEH AND TOFU FLAVOR OPTIONS ARE ENDLESS

Tempeh and tofu are very flexible and take on any flavor you want, making it easy to create simple, healthy meal plans for busy schedules while incorporating the complete high protein source - soy.

Remember: legumes (beans, peas, and lentils) are other high protein options that can be used.

Tempeh is ready to steam, bake, or brown in an intact nonstick skillet as is. For a quick meal, tempeh and pressed tofu can be sliced and marinated for 30 minutes to an hour in beef or chicken flavored bouillon, then seared. For enhanced flavor, soak tempeh in marinade for up to a couple hours before searing. It can also be baked in the oven on parchment paper or a baking mat.

Most people prefer tofu with a more crispy, dense, or fibrous consistency, similar to chicken. This is easily done by freezing, thawing, then squeezing out the water. Once the water is removed, it absorbs marinades well. Thawed tofu cook time is reduced to a few minutes. For people with more time and patience, tofu that has not been frozen can be pressed, then baked or seared, but it takes about 40-45 minutes of bake time for a firmer, crispier consistency. The smaller the tofu pieces are cut, the shorter the cook time and the more palatable it is for new tofu eaters. Combine tofu or tempeh with vegetables and toss them with or drizzle with a sauce like ginger-pineapple, teriyaki, peanut, orange-ginger, barbecue, coconut-curry, nut-butter maple, or a hot sauce over them.

Tempeh, Tofu (or Legumes) Stir Fry Base Recipe

INGREDIENTS
2 cups tempeh or firm tofu, thawed and pressed, cut into bite-sized/small pieces (and/or legumes)

OTHER INGREDIENTS
1 cup whole grain farro, noodles, rice, quinoa, or other grain prepared as recommended (See rice prep.).
4 cups of any bite-sized vegetable combinations like broccoli, sliced carrots, snap peas, chopped bok choy, sliced bell peppers, sliced mushrooms, or sliced onions. Go through your fridge and use up those lovely vegetables.

GARNISH OPTIONS/IDEAS
1 teaspoon sesame seeds, sliced green onions or chives, sliced hot peppers, crushed peanuts, pumpkin seeds, cilantro, or lime wedges

PREPARATION - QUICKEST STOVETOP METHOD
* Prepare grain: For 1 cup rice, rinse and add 6 cups water, cover with a lid, bring to a simmer for 35 minutes, drain well, cover with lid again, and let set on warm burner for about 15 minutes to steam and fluff.
* Prepare a sauce (see options that follow under *Sauces*).
* Bake or sear tempeh or tofu pieces in an oven or nonstick skillet until lightly browned.
* Add 4 cups of any bite-sized vegetables to a large skillet over medium heat with a little water, if needed. Cover and cook vegetables for a minute, then uncover, allowing water to steam off a bit, add sauce, toss, and remove from heat.
* Place grains on plates, top with vegetables and tofu or tempeh, and garnish as desired.

Each sauce recipe makes about 1 cup. Consider doubling the sauce to be used for another night by simply swapping out the vegetables to change it up a bit. Healthy sauces can be used to drizzle over any grain or pasta dish adding flavor and nutritional variety...

Nutty Asian Garlic Sauce

SAUCE INGREDIENTS

1/4 cup low sodium soy sauce or umami sauce
2 tablespoons date paste or syrup, molasses, or maple syrup
2 tablespoons peanut butter or tahini
1 1/2 tablespoons ginger, minced
3 cloves garlic, minced, or 1/8 teaspoon garlic powder
1/2 cup low sodium vegetable broth, or water1/8 teaspoon red pepper flakes, optional
2-3 teaspoons whole grain flour sprinkled over mixture for thickening, while heating, optional
(Consider using ¼ teaspoon xanthan for translucency but remember it takes up to 10 minutes to thicken without heating).

PREPARATION

Prepare sauce by adding the ingredients to a saucepan and simmer to thicken.

Teriyaki Sauce

INGREDIENTS

1/4 cup low sodium soy sauce or umami sauce
1/4 cup water
1/3 cup date paste or syrup, molasses, or honey
1 tablespoon rice vinegar or cider vinegar
1 garlic clove, minced, or 1/8 teaspoon garlic powder
2 teaspoons ginger, minced, or 1/8 teaspoon ginger powder
1/8 teaspoon black pepper, fresh ground
Use whole grain flour sprinkled over mixture for thickening or use
  ¼ teaspoon xanthan for translucency, but remember it takes up to 10 minutes to thicken

PREPARATION

Prepare sauce by adding the ingredients to a saucepan and simmer to thicken.

Ginger Pineapple Sauce

SAUCE INGREDIENTS

1 clove garlic, finely chopped, or 1/8 teaspoon garlic powder

1 tablespoon ginger, finely chopped, or 1/4 teaspoon ginger powder

1/2 cup or 5 pieces of pineapple, fresh or frozen

1/2 cup low sodium vegetable broth, nutritional oil, or water3 tablespoons date sugar, date syrup, molasses, or honey

3 tablespoons low sodium soy sauce or umami sauce

1-2 dashes of cayenne pepper, 1/4 teaspoon red pepper flakes, or 1/2 teaspoon fresh jalapeño peppers minced, optional

2-3 teaspoons whole grain flour sprinkled over mixture for thickening, optional or use
¼ teaspoon xanthan for translucency, but remember it takes up to 10 minutes to thicken

PREPARATION

* Add the ingredients to a blender and blend until smooth.

* Transfer to a saucepan to simmer until thickened.

Lemon-Miso Sauce

Delicious served over broccoli or any grain or vegetables adding a creamy lemony flavor.

SAUCE INGREDIENTS

1 tablespoon light miso paste

1 tablespoon tahini, optional

1 tablespoon date sugar, honey, or maple syrup

2-3 tablespoons fresh blended lemon juice, to taste

1/8 tsp fresh ground pepper, optional

PREPARATION

* Whisk by hand or add the ingredients to a blender and blend until smooth.

Cumin Lime Sauce

Server over any salad, grains, rice, or vegeatables to add fresh flavor with zing.

INGREDIENTS

2 tablespoons red onion, finely chopped or minced, optional

2 cloves garlic, minced

1/3 cup lime juice

1 tablespoon honey

2 teaspoons light miso slurry, optional

1 teaspoon cumin

2 tablespoons cilantro, finely chopped

2 tablespoons seaweed (nori, alaria) finely chopped or torn in pieces

PREPARATION

* Combine all ingredients and toss together.

Pasta Dishes

Spaghetti and "Meatballs"

Lasagna

Macaroni and Cheese

Creamy Pasta with Cauliflower Cream Sauce

Lentils Bolognese Pasta

Daily Dozen Spaghetti and "Meatballs"

Loaded with nutrients, this recipe includes food from all of Dr. Greger's Daily Dozen nutrient recommendations checklist. Some of these ingredients may seem strange for a spaghetti sauce, but you will be quite impressed with the flavor. There is a variety of nondairy, eggless, and gluten-free pasta options available today, made from healthy, whole plant sources like lentils, chickpeas, black beans, beets, and cauliflower. If you haven't tried spaghetti squash yet, it is a delicious healthy noodle option with a fresh crunch that our family absolutely loves.

1 box whole grain, legume, or vegetable pasta

INGREDIENTS

1 cup carrots, sliced, then finely chopped

1 cup onion, chopped or sliced

4 cloves garlic, pressed, minced, or sliced

2 cups mushrooms, portobello or shiitake, chopped or sliced

1 bell pepper, chopped or sliced

1 cup kale, collards, chard, arugula, or spinach, chopped

1/4 cup concord grapes, cherries, or raisins, chopped

1/4 cup date paste, date sugar, apple sauce, prunes, or pears

2 tablespoons flaxseeds, crushed

2 tablespoons hempseeds, pumpkin seeds, chia seeds, or nuts

4 cups of low sodium vegetable stock or water

2 15-ounce cans diced tomatoes

28-42 ounces of tomatoes, crushed

1 12-ounce jar tomato paste

4 bay leaves

1 tablespoons Italian seasoning

2 teaspoons fennel, partially crushed, mortar and pestle or coffee grinder work well (sausage flavor)

1 teaspoon turmeric

1/4 cup nutritional yeast

1/2 teaspoon ground black pepper or 1/4 teaspoon cayenne pepper or red pepper flakes

2-3 tablespoons low sodium soy sauce or dark miso paste slurry, adjust to taste

1-2 cups black beans or tempeh, roughly chopped, crumbled, or chopped

GARNISHES AND SIDES

Fresh basil or parsley, whole grain garlic bread, and a side salad

PREPARATION

* Add carrots to a food processor and chop into small pieces. Chop or slice remaining INGREDIENTS either in the processor or by hand.

* Transfer in batches to a large non-stick pot over medium heat or a crockpot.

* Add remaining ingredients and bring to a simmer.

* Reduce heat to simmer or low for about 6 hours for richest flavor, stirring regularly. When using a gas cooktop, bring to a simmer while stirring, then turn off heat and repeat every hour or so to prevent hanging over the stove all day.

* Prepare pasta, a salad, and whole grain garlic bread.

* Top noodles with sauce, meatballs (See recipe), nondairy mozzarella, and fresh basil leaves.

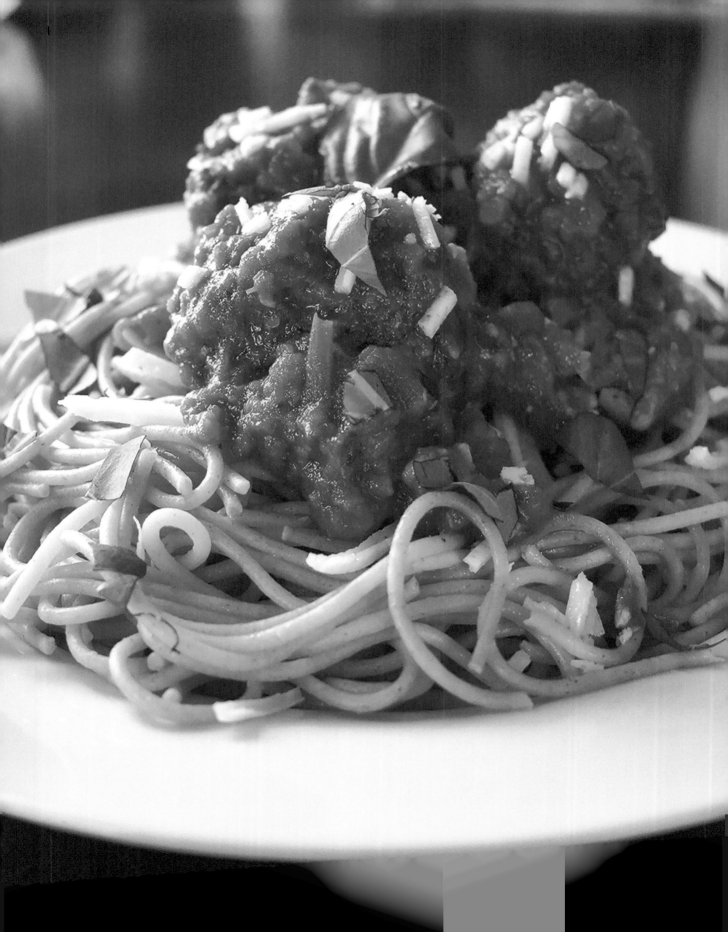

Macaroni and Cheese

This nondairy cheese sauce can also be used as a cheese dip or as a topping for baked potatoes and steamed broccoli. Save leftovers for a week in refrigerator or freeze it to enjoy within a month. Can also bake macaroni as a casserole with broccoli stirred in, adding whole grain panko/breadcrumb topping.

PASTA

8 ounces whole grain or vegetable pasta (macaroni elbows)
Broccoli or peas, fresh or frozen

STEAMED VEGETABLE INGREDIENTS

1/3 cup raw cashews, hemp seeds, or cauliflower (bite sized pieces)
1/2 cup white beans, or potatoes (bite-sized pieces)
1/4 cup carrots (thin slices) or butternut squash
1/4 cup mild onion, chopped
1 cup low sodium vegetable broth or water

OTHER INGREDIENTS

2 teaspoons lemon juice
1/4 cup nutritional yeast
1/2 teaspoon stone ground mustard or Dijon, optional
1/2 teaspoon garlic powder
1/4 teaspoon turmeric
1/4 - 1/2 teaspoon paprika (smoked paprika adds a nice flavor)
1-2 pinches cayenne pepper, optional
2 tablespoons light miso paste
4-5 low sodium green olives or 1/2 teaspoon salt + 1 teaspoon soy powder or some soybeans/tempeh

PREPARATION

* Begin to prepare macaroni pasta and plan preparation of broccoli, peas, or side salad.

* Meanwhile, place STEAMED VEGETABLE INGREDIENTS in a saucepan, cover with a lid, bring to a simmer for 5-10 minutes, turn off heat, allowing them to steam for 15 minutes more (do not drain.)

* Add OTHER INGREDIENTS to the blender and blend until creamy.

* Add STEAMED VEGETABLE INGREDIENTS to the blender, blend until creamy, then transfer back to the saucepan. Adjust creaminess with broth or water.

* Heat and stir sauce over medium heat and combine about half of the sauce with the drained pasta.

* *If baking,* stir in uncooked bite-sized broccoli or peas, transfer to a 9 x 9 inch or high side 8 x 8-inch baking dish, sprinkle with whole grain bread crumbs, panko, or nondairy parmesan cheese and paprika. Bake on center rack until golden brown for 15-20 minutes.

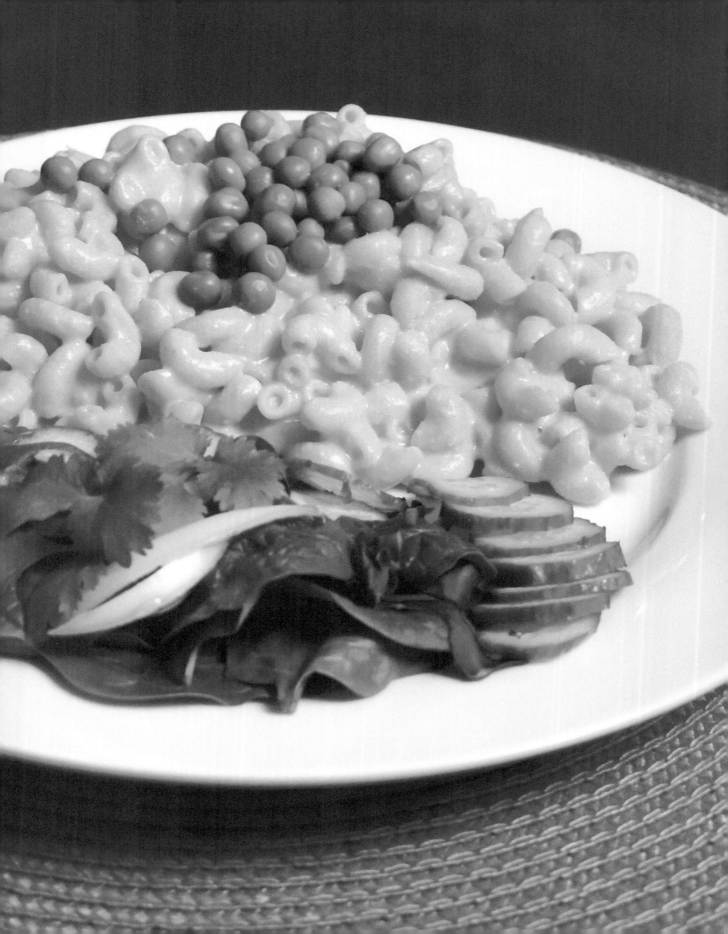

Creamy Pasta with Cauliflower Cream Sauce

This dish is a definite family pleaser. You don't have to feel guilty about having seconds with food this healthy, but the first dish will most likely satisfy you. Consider enjoying with peas, carrots, broccoli, asparagus, roasted vegetables, or *King Oyster Mushroom Scallops* (See recipe).

INGREDIENTS

1 pound or 1 box of whole grain or vegetable pasta

CASHEW CAULIFLOWER SAUCE INGREDIENTS

1/2 cup mild onion, sliced or chopped
2-3 cloves of garlic, sliced or minced
1/2 cup raw cashews, white beans, raw hempseeds, or 1/3 cup lowfat coconut milk
1 cup cauliflower, cut into pieces
1 cup low sodium vegetable stock, broth, or water

OTHER SAUCE INGREDIENTS

1 cup plain nondairy unsweetened milk, broth, or water
1/4 cup nutritional yeast
2 teaspoons lemon juice
2 tablespoons light miso paste slurry
1/8 teaspoon crushed red pepper flakes or 2 pinches cayenne, optional

GARNISH OPTIONS

Fresh ground black pepper to taste, chopped basil, parsley, hot peppers, or nondairy parmesan cheese

PREPARATION

* Add onion and garlic to a saucepan over medium heat and cook until lightly browned/caramelized.

* Add cashews, cauliflower, and broth to the saucepan, cover with a lid, and simmer for 10 minutes.

* Remove from heat and allow to set 15 minutes more to soak. Do not drain.

* Meanwhile, prepare pasta in another pot, drain, and return to pot.

* Transfer undrained cashews and cauliflower and OTHER SAUCE INGREDIENTS to a blender and process until creamy.

* Pour desired amount of sauce over pasta, and heat through.

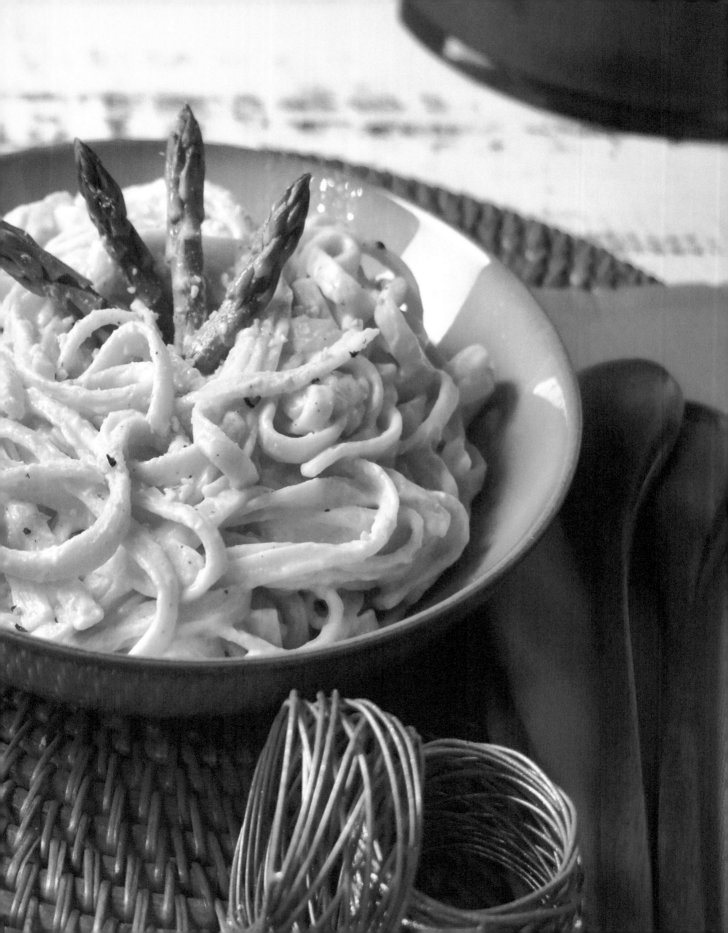

Lasagna

Finding healthy pre-made cheese that tastes good can be a challenge, but you *can* make your own. Lasagna is already known as a time-consuming process, so if you plan to make your own cheese (plant-based parmesan, ricotta, or mozzarella), consider doing it a day ahead.

SAUCE INGREDIENTS - Roughly chop following ingredients to resemble beef/sausage crumbles

2 medium carrots, chopped (Consider using a food processor for carrots separately)

2 cups mushrooms, chopped

1/2 large onion, chopped

1/2 bell pepper, chopped

2-3 cloves garlic, minced or ¼ teaspoon garlic powder

1 ½ - 2 cups black beans and/or tempeh, roughly crumbled by hand

1/4 cup date paste, date sugar, chopped raisins, or maple syrup

1 tablespoon Italian seasoning

1 teaspoon dried basil

1 teaspoon oregano

2-3 teaspoons fennel seeds, semicrushed (sausage flavor)

1 teaspoon fresh ground pepper

1/4-1/2 cup low sodium soy sauce, dark miso paste slurry, or 1/2 teaspoon salt (tempeh helps buffer)

1 cup or 1 6-oz can cup tomato paste

1 cup petite diced tomatoes

1 ½ cups crushed tomato or purée

1/4 cup nutritional yeast

1 tablespoon beef bouillon, optional (See recipe)

OTHER INGREDIENTS

1 cup plant-based *Parmesan Cheese* (See recipe)

1 ½ cups plant-based *Ricotta Cheese* (See recipe) and make ahead

2-4 cups leafy greens, chopped

2 zucchini, sliced lengthwise, 1/4 inch thick, optional

10-12 lasagna noodles, whole grain or vegetable pasta—just soak in warm water for about 10 minutes (No need to boil)

PREPARATION

* Preheat oven to 350°F.

* Place the chopped carrots, mushrooms, onion, bell pepper, and garlic in a large nonstick pot over medium heat and simmer until softened or lightly browned.

* Add remaining *INGREDIENTS,* cover, and return to a simmer for 30 more minutes.

* If using zucchini as a layer, lay out zucchini slices on a parchment lined baking sheet or baking mat and bake for 10-15 minutes, watching carefully until lightly browned.

* To assemble, spread a thin layer of SAUCE INGREDIENTS in the bottom of a 9 x 13 inch baking dish and arrange a layer of noodles on top. Spread half of the ricotta mixture over the noodles.

* Add a thin layer of each—chopped greens, zucchini, sauce, noodles, ricotta, chopped greens, zucchini, sauce—and add a light layer of parmesan.

* Bake in preheated oven for 25-30 minutes.

* After baking, top with a light sprinkling of plant-based parmesan cheese and fresh parsley or green onions for presentation.

* Cool for 15 minutes before serving. Serve with salad and whole grain garlic bread.

* Wrap and freeze leftovers in serving size portions..

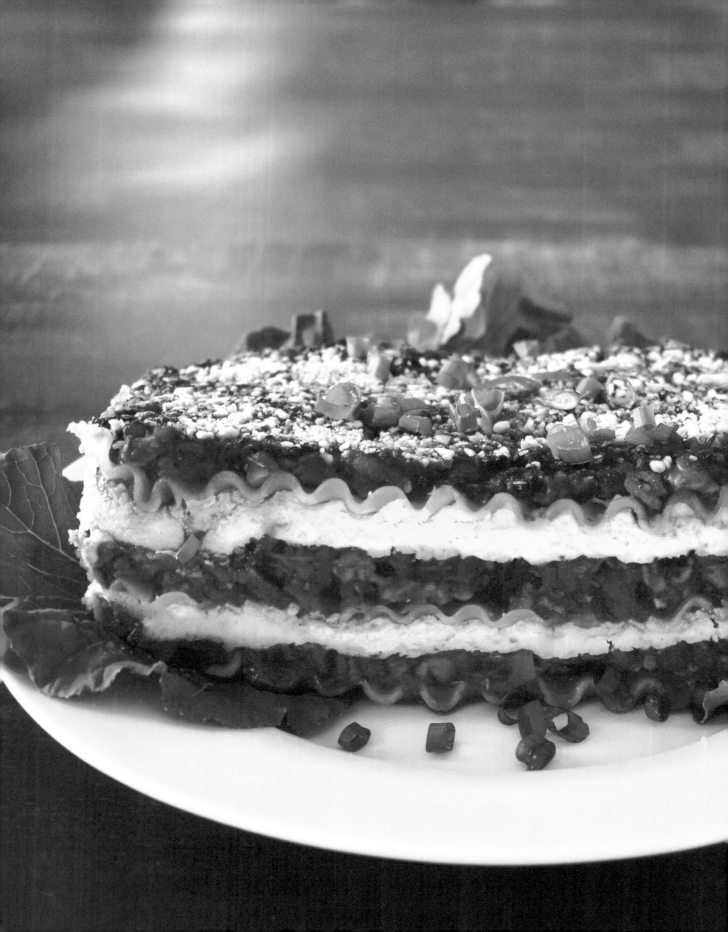

Lentils Bolognese Pasta

PASTA

1 pound/box of whole grain or vegetable pasta

SAUTÉ INGREDIENTS—consider chopping the following vegetables in a food processor

1 cup onion, chopped

1 cup bell pepper, chopped

1 celery stalk, chopped or thinly sliced

1 cup carrots, finely chopped

3 cloves garlic, minced or sliced

1 cup mushrooms, chopped

1 tablespoon (porcini) mushroom powder, optional

1/4 cup low sodium vegetable broth or water

OTHER INGREDIENTS

2 cups low sodium vegetable stock, broth, or water

1 cup green or brown lentils, rinsed well

1/2 cup whole grains, cooked or 1/2 cup tempeh, crumbled

2 cups petite diced tomatoes, with juice

1/3 cup tomato paste or 1/3 cup sundried tomatoes, chopped

1 tablespoon Italian seasoning

1 teaspoon smoked paprika or 1/2 teaspoon liquid smoke

1 teaspoon basil

1 tablespoon balsamic vinegar

3 tablespoons raisins or dates, chopped

1/2 teaspoon red pepper flakes or fresh ground black pepper

1/4 cup nondairy parmesan cheese

1-2 tablespoons miso paste slurry

PREPARATION

* Chop SAUTÉ VEGETABLES in a food processor, transfer to a large pot over medium heat and cook until onions become tender.

* Add 2 cups stock/broth, lentils, grains/tempeh, and tomatoes, cover with a lid, simmer for 30 minutes, then remove from heat.

* Add remaining ingredients except for miso and "parmesan" and simmer for 20 minutes more.

* Allow to cool for 15 minutes, then add miso and parmesan.

* Meanwhile, in another pot, cook pasta until al denté, then drain and return to pot with a ladle of sauce stirred into it.

* Place a ladle full over each plate of pasta, and garnish with fresh parsley or basil.

* Serve with a side salad and whole grain garlic bread.

Side Dishes

Yellow Rice and Beans

Unfried Rice

Simple Baked Beans

Apple Sauce, Homemade

Cumin Lime Slaw

Coleslaw and Dressing

Unfried French Fries

Yellow Rice and Beans

Consider serving this with tacos, burritos, a side salad, tempeh, or tofu.

RICE INGREDIENTS

1 cup basmati or jasmine rice, rinsed well
1/4 cup hot vegetable broth or water
1/2 teaspoon black pepper
1/4 teaspoon cumin, ground
1/2 teaspoon turmeric, ground
1 tablespoon light miso paste slurry or
1/4 teaspoon salt + 1/2 teaspoon soy powder

SAUTÉ INGREDIENTS

1/4 cup low sodium vegetable broth, or water
1 cup chopped onion
1 bell pepper, chopped, any color
1 jalapeño pepper, finely chopped
2 garlic cloves, minced
2 cups or 1 can black beans
1 teaspoon fennel, crushed

GARNISHI OPTIONS

2 cups cherry tomatoes, sliced, 1/2 cup cilantro
or salsa

PREPARATION

* Cook rice over medium heat, cover with a lid, bring to a simmer for 35 minutes, drain well, cover with lid again, and let set on warm burner for about 15 minutes more.

* Combine other RICE INGREDIENTS in a small bowl or saucepan, pour over rice, and stir to combine.

* Add SAUTÉ INGREDIENTS to a nonstick skillet, cook on medium heat until onion is softened, then combine with rice.

* Place rice and beans on each plate and garnish with tomatoes, cilantro, or salsa.

Unfried Rice

This pairs well with a mixed greens salad or an Asian salad topped with sesame ginger dressing (See recipe).

RICE PREPARATION

2 cups whole short grain rice, cooked in 10 cups of water, simmered for 35 minutes, drained well, then covered with a lid and set on warm burner to steam 10 minutes more.

FLAVOR OPTIONS

For "chicken fried rice," use 1/2 block of tempeh or previously frozen firm tofu, thawed, pressed, torn, and soaked in 1 cup vegetable chickenless bouillon sautéed or baked 20 minutes, or try 2 cups precooked chickpeas, rinsed and sautéed, with 1 tablespoon vegetable chickenless bouillon.

For "egg fried rice," use 1/2 block previously frozen silken tofu, thawed, pressed, crumbled, sautéed, and coated with 1 teaspoon turmeric and 1 teaspoon kala namak (to taste/health).

BASE INGREDIENTS

2 cups carrots, chopped
1 cup sweet onion, chopped
4 cloves garlic, minced or sliced
1 cup frozen or fresh peas
3-4 tablespoons low sodium soy sauce
1 tablespoon nutritional yeast or vegetable
  "chicken" bouillon, (See recipe) adjust to taste

GARNISH OPTIONS

2 tablespoons green onions, chopped

1 teaspoon sesame seeds

PREPARATION

* Cook rice per recommendation

* Over medium heat, add carrots and onions to a large skillet and cook for about 5 minutes.

* Add remaining BASE INGREDIENTS, cover with a lid, and cook for 5-8 minutes more.

* Add FLAVOR OPTION to skillet and heat through.

* Top with green onions and sesame seeds.

Simple Baked Beans

1 cup onion, sliced or chopped, optional

1/2 cup bell pepper, chopped, optional

1/4 cup low sodium vegetable stock or water

OTHER INGREDIENTS

2-4 cups pinto beans, kidney beans, or navy beans, cooked and rinsed

1/2 cup low sodium vegetable stock or water

1/2 cup organic ketchup (no fructose corn syrup)

1/4 cup date sugar, date syrup, apple sauce, or maple syrup, to taste/health

1 tablespoon molasses

1/2 teaspoon dry mustard or 2 teaspoons whole grain mustard

1 tablespoon plant-based Worcestershire sauce or cider vinegar

1 teaspoon smoked paprika

1 tablespoon jalapeño peppers, minced or 1/4 teaspoon black pepper, optional

PREPARATION

* Cook on the stovetop or bake as a casserole.

* Stovetop, add SAUTÉ INGREDIENTS over medium heat and cook until onions are softened or caramelized, then add OTHER INGREDIENTS, bring to a simmer to cook for another 15 minutes, stirring occasionally. Add stock or water as needed.

* If using a casserole or baking dish, combine all ingredients in a mixing bowl, pour into casserole dish, and bake for 30 minutes.

Homemade Applesauce

INGREDIENTS

6 medium apples, peel and cut into wedges

1/2 cup water

2 tablespoons date sugar or pure maple syrup, optional

1 tablespoon lemon juice

1/2 teaspoon cinnamon, optional

1/4 teaspoon vanilla bean powder, paste, or extract, optional

PREPARATION

Add all ingredients to a medium-sized pot over medium heat, bring to a short boil, reduce heat to simmer, cover, and cook 15-20 minutes, stirring occasionally.

Cumin Lime Slaw

INGREDIENTS

2 cups cabbage, thinly sliced

1/4 cup red onion, chopped or thinly sliced

1-2 cloves garlic, minced

1/4 cup lime juice

2 teaspoons honey

2 teaspoons light miso slurry, optional

1 teaspoon cumin

1/4 cup cilantro

2 tablespoons seaweed (nori, alaria) finely chopped

PREPARATION

* Combine all ingredients and toss together.

Coleslaw

INGREDIENTS
3-4 cups cabbage, finely shredded
1/2 cup carrots, finely shredded
2 tablespoons onion, minced

Coleslaw Dressing

2 tablespoons rice wine vinegar or cider vinegar
4 tablespoons honey or date syrup
1/2 teaspoon dry mustard powder or 1 teaspoon ground mustard
1 tablespoon light miso paste slurry
1/2 teaspoon celery seed
3/4 cup plant-based mayonnaise

PREPARATION
Combine dressing in a small bowl and mix into Coleslaw.

Unfried French Fries

Potato slices, wedges, or strips crisp up beautifully in an air fryer. Baking them in an oven takes longer and they usually don't crisp up as well. Try organic or homemade ketchup to avoid high fructose corn syrup.

INGREDIENTS
3 medium potatoes, sliced into fry strips
1 tablespoon light miso paste slurry or 1/4 teaspoon salt + soy powder, optional
1 teaspoon garlic, optional
1/4 teaspoon black pepper, optional
1 tablespoon nondairy parmesan cheese, optional (See recipe)
1 tablespoon fresh parsley, dill, or rosemary, finely chopped, optional
1 teaspoon nutritional yeast, optional

INSTRUCTIONS

* Use an air fryer with the settings and directions provided or

* Preheat oven to 400°F. Prepare a nonstick baking mat or a baking sheet with parchment paper.

* In a large mixing bowl, combine your choice of ingredients, add sliced potatoes, toss to coat and spread out in a single layer on a baking sheet.

* Bake potatoes for 6-15 minutes, depending on size of slices. Watch for light browning on edges, turn over and cook until lightly browned on edges again.

Salads

Cucumber Bean Fiesta Salad

Greens with Orange Balsamic Dressing

Greek Quinoa Salad

Sweet Potato Brussel Sprouts Salad

Broccoli Slaw

Potato Salad, Homestyle

Potato Salad, Southern Style

Cucumber Bean Fiesta Salad or Dip

The nice thing about this is that you just get out a big bowl and throw it all in there. Easy to make and is extremely popular! This is a great dish to double up on for a party and for your family who will be circling over while you are preparing it. Serve as a salad with the Strawberry Blush Wine Vinaigrette Dressing (See recipe) or a balsamic dressing. Serve over leafy greens or enjoy as a salsa dip.

INGREDIENTS

2-3 avocados, small cubes
4 cups or 2 cans of beans (we use half black and half white beans)
1 large bell pepper, chopped (any color)
1/2-1 cup chopped cilantro
3 cloves garlic
1/2 cup purple or sweet onion
2 cups tomatoes (cherry or grape), sliced in half or diced
1-2 cups cucumber, cubed
1 can corn or 2 cups frozen, cooked (grilled or roasted is a tasty option)
1-2 medium fresh jalapeño or serrano peppers, finely chopped, optional for some
2 teaspoons lime juice, drizzled over avocados

PREPARATION

* Cut up avocado and place in a small bowl. Drizzle with lime juice.

* In a large bowl combine remaining ingredients.

* Add some vinaigrette or balsamic dressing.

* Gently fold avocado into the vegetable mix.

* Garnish with pumpkin seeds or nondairy feta, optional.

Greens with Orange Balsamic Dressing

This simple sauce can help increase your dark leafy greens intake. Some favorite ways to serve it are with beets, onions, and wilted beet greens or any leafy greens, onion, and orange slices or other fruit.

DRESSING INGREDIENTS

1 tablespoon date sugar, date syrup, maple syrup, or honey
1/4 cup blended orange juice
2 tablespoons balsamic vinaigrette
1 teaspoon ground mustard
1 teaspoon tahini or gelled flax seed
  Pepper to taste

PREPARATION

* Combine dressing ingredients in a small bowl. Wash beets, remove stem and root, slice into 1/2-3/4 inch wedges, wrap in foil, and bake in 400 degree oven for 30 minutes or steam them in a saucepan. When softened, pour dressing into skillet over medium heat, reduce liquid for a few minutes, add onions and beet greens and cook until wilted.

Greek Quinoa Salad

INGREDIENTS

1 cup quinoa

DRESSING INGREDIENTS

1/4 cup lemon juice, red wine vinegar, rice wine vinegar, or white balsamic

1 tablespoon light miso paste slurry or 2 teaspoons low sodium soy sauce

1/3 cup nutritional oil (See recipe)

2 cloves garlic, minced or pressed or ¼ teaspoon powdered

1/2 teaspoon oregano, dried

1/2 teaspoon basil, dried

1/2 teaspoon Dijon mustard

1/4 teaspoon black pepper, fresh ground

REMAINING INGREDIENTS

1 cup cherry tomatoes, halved

1/3 cup kalamata or black olives, pitted

1/2-1 yellow bell pepper, chopped

1/4 cup parsley

1/2 teaspoon fresh ground black pepper

1/4 cup red onion, thinly sliced or diced

1 cucumber, diced

GARNISH

1/4 cup green onions, thinly sliced plant-based feta or a few more low sodium olives.

PREPARATION

* Combine DRESSING INGREDIENTS and allow the flavors to meld.

* Rinse quinoa and combine with two cups of low sodium vegetable stock, broth, or water in a saucepan, bring to a short boil, cover with a lid, and reduce to simmer for 25 minutes.

* Transfer quinoa to a mixing bowl. Fluff with a fork to cool a bit.

* Add REMAINING INGREDIENTS and toss to combine with the dressing.

* Top with additional fresh parsley, olives, or veggie feta or kalamata olives.

Sweet Potato Brussel Sprouts Salad

VEGETABLES

2 cups fresh kale or spinach, uncooked, chopped
4 cups sweet potatoes, cut into 3/4-inch cubes
3 cups Brussels sprouts, 1/4-inch slices
1 medium red onion, sliced into 1/4-inch wedges
1 bell pepper, chopped or sliced

DRESSING INGREDIENTS

2 teaspoons fresh oregano or 1/2 teaspoon dry
2 teaspoons low sodium soy sauce
1/2 cup nutritional oil (See recipe)
1 tablespoon nutritional yeast
1 tablespoon flaxseeds, crushed
1/4 cup balsamic vinaigrette
2 teaspoons date syrup or pure maple syrup
2 teaspoons ground pepper

PREPARATION

* Preheat oven to 400°F. Place portions of massaged kale on individual serving plates.
* Combine VEGETABLES in a large mixing bowl.
* Combine DRESSING INGREDIENTS in a small bowl or pitcher, and drizzle about 1/4 cup over the vegetables and toss to mix.
* Spread vegetables out on a parchment sheet or nonstick baking mat.
* Bake for about 30 minutes, turning over after halfway through cooking.
* Place VEGETABLES on kale, drizzle more dressing over the salad, and garnish with pumpkin seeds, pomegranate seeds, or raisins.

Broccoli Slaw

INGREDIENTS

3 cups broccoli slaw (finely shredded broccoli), food processor shred blade works well
3/4 cup carrots, shredded
3/4 cup red cabbage, thinly sliced or shredded
1 cup raisins, organic craisins (no high fructose corn syrup), grapes, or apples, chopped or cut into small pieces
1/4 cup green or red onion, thinly sliced or chopped

DRESSSING INGREDIENTS

1/2 cup nutritional oil (See recipe)
2 teaspoons flax, chia seeds, or ¼ teaspoon xanthan powder to thicken.
3 tablespoons apple cider vinegar
1 1/4 teaspoon dry mustard powder
1/4 cup pure honey or maple syrup

1 tablespoon miso paste slurry
1/2 avocado, ripe
3 tablespoons oats
3/4 teaspoon celery seed
1/2 teaspoon black pepper

GARNISH

3 tablespoons pumpkin seeds
3 tablespoons almonds, slivered

PREPARATION

* In a food processor, shred broccoli, carrots, and cabbage and transfer to a large bowl. Add raisins, grapes, apples, and onions to the bowl and toss to mix.
* In a blender or food processor, add DRESSING INGREDIENTS and blend until creamy.
* Garnish with pumpkin seeds and/or almonds.

Potato Salad, Homestyle

Similar to pototo salad popular at cookouts in western Pennsylvania. Another very easy potato salad that takes no time to prepare is listed below.

5-6 potatoes, red potatoes or Yukon Gold

DRESSING INGREDIENTS
1/2 cup plant-based mayonnaise (See recipe)
1/2 block soft tofu
2-3 dashes kala namak (egg flavor)
1 dash of turmeric
1 tablespoon cider vinegar
1 tablespoon light miso paste
1 tablespoon mustard

OTHER DRESSING INGREDIENTS
1/2-1 teaspoon celery seeds
1/4 cup fresh dill, chopped, or 1 teaspoon dried
1/4 cup sweet pickle relish

ADDITONAL INGREDIENTS
1 red, orange, or green bell pepper, chopped
1/2 cup onion, finely chopped
1/4 cup celery, finely chopped
1/4 teaspoon black pepper, fresh ground
1/4-1/2 teaspoon paprika, sprinkled over potato salad

PREPARATION

* Remove eyes and cut the potatoes into 1/2-inch cubes and place them in a large pot with enough stock, broth, or water to cover.

* Bring to a boil, reduce heat to medium, and cook uncovered for about 10 minutes until nearly done. Check with a knife tip (don't overcook). Drain water from potatoes and set aside to cool.

* In a food processor, add DRESSING INGREDIENTS and blend until creamy. Then add OTHER DRESSING INGREDIENTS to food processor and pulse 2 or 3 times to gently combine, then transfer to a large bowl with the potatoes.

* Add ADDITIONAL INGREDIENTS except for paprika, stir to combine, and sprinkle with paprika.

Potato Salad, Southern Style

One of the tastiest potato salads you can whip up in a jiffy. Inspired by Ann Crile Esselstyn's friend, Jan, in Ann's cookbook *The Prevent and Reverse Heart Disease Cookbook*, which I highly recommend!

INGREDIENTS
3-4 medium potatoes, cooked al denté and cooled
1-2 stalks of celery, finely chopped
1/2 cup onion or shallots, finely chopped
1/3 cup unsweetened, plain apple sauce
1/4 cup mustard (whole ground or Dijon)
2 teaspoons cider vinegar
1-2 tablespoons chopped fresh dill or 1/2 teaspoon dried dill
1/4 cup dill or sweet relish (or chopped pickles)

PREPARATION

* Combine cooked potatoes with celery and onion.

* Combine apple sauce, mustard, 1/2 of the dill, relish, and vinegar.

* Mix together and top with remaining dill, pepper, and any desired seasoning like pepper, paprika, or Salt Reduction Seasoning (See recipe).

Dressings, Sauces, and Condiments

Nutritional Oil

Honey Dijon Vinaigrette

Balsamic Vinaigrette Dressing

Simple Vinaigrette Dressing

Sesame Ginger Dressing

Strawberry Blush Wine Vinaigrette

Cilantro Lime Dressing

Berry Balsamic Vinaigrette

Ranch Dressing

Ketchup

Barbecue Sauce

Mayonnaise

Sour Cream

Red Curry Paste

Nutritional Oil

Dr. Esselstyn is famously known for saying "NO OIL". He absolutely knows what it takes to reverse heart disease. He dedicated his life to his heart patients doing just that. Use this as a healthy oil replacement in your homemade salad dressings and in any other recipes calling for oil.

INGREDIENTS

1 cup warm water
1 teaspoon nutritional yeast, to taste
1 teaspoon light miso paste

THICKENING INGREDIENT OPTIONS

1/4 teaspoon xanthan powder, 1 tablespoon crushed flaxseed (heart healthy), or 2 teaspoons tahini, optional (xanthan powder and flaxseed take 5-10 minutes to thicken)

PREPARATION

Add ingredients to a blender and blend well for 30 seconds to a minute (for flaxseed) until smooth.

Honey Dijon Vinaigrette

Try this drizzled over roasted beets and lightly sautéed beet greens topped with walnuts and pumpkin seeds.

INGREDIENTS

1/4 cup nutritional oil (See recipe)
2 tablespoons Dijon mustard
2 tablespoon cider vinegar or red wine vinegar
1 tablespoon honey, date syrup, or maple syrup
1 clove garlic or 1/4 teaspoon garlic powder
1 tablespoon finely chopped onion or 1/4 teaspoon dried onion
1 teaspoon light miso paste
pepper to taste

PREPARATION

Whisk or blend all ingredients to to a creamy consistency.

Balsamic Vinaigrette Dressing

INGREDIENTS

1/2 cup nutritional oil
¼ cup balsamic vinegar
1-2 teaspoons date syrup, maple syrup, or honey
1 teaspoon Dijon mustard
1 shallot/onion, minced
1 clove garlic, minced
1-2 teaspoons of white miso paste
1/8 teaspoon of fresh ground pepper

PREPARATION

Add ingredients to a blender to blend and let set for 10 minutes to thicken.

Simple Vinaigrette Dressing

INGREDIENTS
1/3 cup cider vinegar
1/3 cup nutritional oil (See recipe)
1 tsp Dijon mustard or 1/2 teaspoon dry mustard
1 tablespoon honey, date paste, or maple syrup
1 tablespoon light miso paste (or 1/2 teaspoon natural salt + 1 teaspoon soy powder,
   soybeans, or tempeh)
1 teaspoon chia seeds or flaxseeds, optional for thickening

PREPARATION
Combine ingredients in a blender and blend until smooth.

Sesame Ginger Dressing

INGREDIENTS
6 tablespoons rice wine vinegar
1/2 cup nutritional oil (See recipe)
2 tablespoons honey, maple syrup, or date syrup
2 tablespoons low sodium soy sauce
2 tablespoons ginger root, grated or chopped
1/4 cup tahini (sesame) or nut butter

PREPARATION
Combine ingredients in a blender on high for about a minute.

Strawberry Blush Wine Vinaigrette

This dressing is nice over a spinach salad with strawberries, blueberries, and thinly sliced purple onions.
Consider combining ingredients with a strawberry and some onion and blend to a creamy dressing.

INGREDIENTS
1/4 cup nutritional oil (See recipe)
1/4-1/3 cup honey, maple syrup, or date sugar
1/4 cup red wine vinegar
1 tablespoon light miso paste (or 1/2 teaspoon natural salt + 3/4 teaspoon soy powder, soybeans/tempeh)
1/4 teaspoon garlic powder
1/4 teaspoon onion powder
2-3 pinches cayenne powder

PREPARATION
Combine ingredients in a blender and blend until smooth.

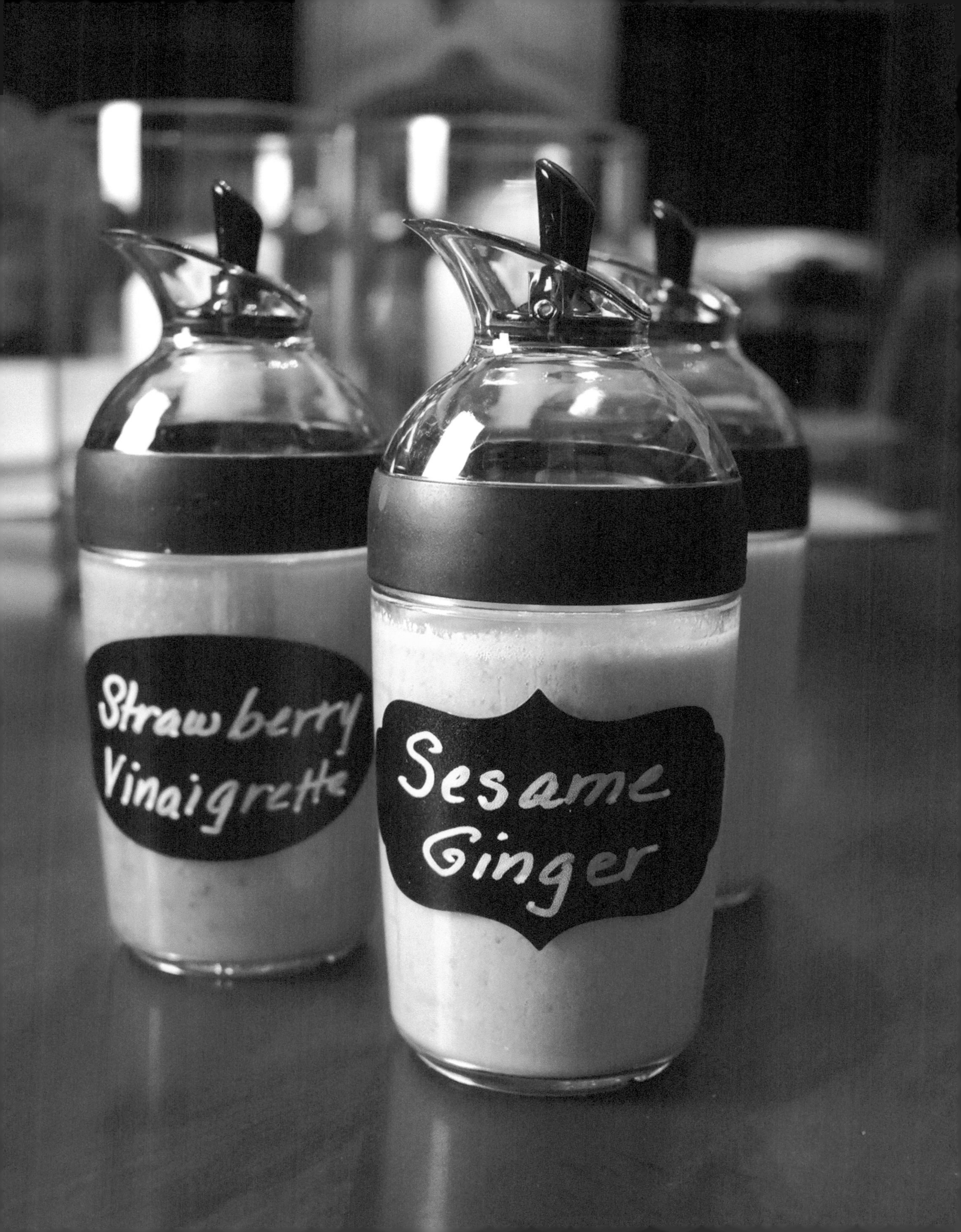
Strawberry
Vinaigrette
Sesame
Ginger

Cilantro Lime Dressing

This dressing works well on tacos and wraps, and on burgers and salads.

INGREDIENTS
1/3 cup rice vinegar
3/4 cup nutritional oil (See recipe)
1 cup cilantro
2 teaspoons honey or maple syrup
1/2 jalapeño pepper, sliced
1 garlic clove, pressed or sliced
1/4 cup blended lime juice
1 tablespoon light miso paste

PREPARATION
Add all ingredients to a blender, and blend to desired creaminess.

Berry Balsamic Vinaigrette

A simple colorful treat to drizzle over your salads, grain bowls, or other dish needing some flavor.

INGREDIENTS
1 cup berries or fruit (blueberries, strawberries, raspberries, mango, etc.)
1/4 cup balsamic or cider vinegar
1/2 cup nutritional oil (See recipe) or 1/2 cup water + 1/2 tsp nutritional yeast + 1/2 tsp miso paste + 1/8
   teaspoon xanthan powder
1-2 tablespoons date paste or honey
1 tablespoons lemon juiced/blended or whole grain mustard
Pepper to taste

PREPARATION
Add ingredients to a blender to blend and let set for 10 minutes to thicken.

Ranch Dressing

INGREDIENTS
1/2 cup raw cashews, 1/2 cup creamed
   cauliflower, or 1/4 cup powdered oats plus
   1/4 cup water
1/2 block tofu, unfrozen
1 tablespoon lemon juice or cider vinegar
2 cloves garlic, minced or pressed, or 1/2
   teaspoon garlic powder
2 teaspoons light miso paste
1/4 teaspoon black pepper, fresh ground
2 tablespoons red onion, minced or chopped, or
   1/4 teaspoon onion powder

1 teaspoon whole grain mustard
1 teaspoon nutritional yeast
1/2 teaspoon fresh parsley or pinch of dried
1 tablespoon fresh dill or 1/2 teaspoon dried

PREPARATION
* Combine all ingredients in a blender except for
   parsley and dill, and blend until smooth.
* Add parsley and dill and pulse 2-3 times to
   combine.
* Refrigerate for an hour to allow flavors to
   meld.

Ketchup

Many commercial ketchups contain high fructose corn syrup and a lot of salt. This recipe gives you control over what goes into yours.

INGREDIENTS

6-ounce can tomato paste
1/2 cup apple cider vinegar or white vinegar
1/4-1/2 cup water, adjust consistency
1/4 teaspoon dry ground mustard
1 tablespoon miso paste or 2 teaspoons low sodium soy sauce
   (or 1/2 teaspoon salt + 1 teaspoon soy powder)
1/4 teaspoon onion powder
1/8 teaspoon garlic powder
1 pinch cayenne pepper
2-3 tablespoons date paste, honey, or maple syrup, to taste/health

PREPARATION

Combine all ingredients in a saucepan, stirring frequently. Bring to a brief boil and reduce heat to simmer for 15-20 minutes. Taste to adjust for desired flavor.

Barbecue Sauce

INGREDIENTS

1 cup organic ketchup
2-3 tablespoons pure maple syrup, date syrup, or honey
1 tablespoon molasses
1 tablespoon low sodium soy sauce
1/2 teaspoon onion powder
1/2 cup balsamic or apple cider vinegar
2 garlic cloves, pressed or minced
1 teaspoon black pepper, ground, or 1/4 teaspoon cayenne pepper
1 tablespoon miso paste, add after cooking

PREPARATION

In a saucepan, combine all sauce ingredients, bring to short boil over medium heat, reduce and simmer for about 15 minutes.

Mayonnaise

It is difficult to find a plant-based, storebought mayonnaise brand that meets health and taste standards. To eliminate egg, genetically modified ingredients, trans fats, and chemical preservatives, consider making it at home. These ingredients make about 1 1/4 cups and lasts for about a week in the refrigerator.

INGREDIENTS

1/4 cup raw cashews (simmered and soaked 30 minutes) or raw hemp seeds
3/4 block or 1 ½ cups plain unfrozen firm tofu or 1 ½ cups cauliflower, steamed/cooked
1 tablespoon lemon juice
2 tablespoons cider vinegar or rice vinegar
1 teaspoonsDijon mustard
1/2 teaspoon onion powder
1/4 teaspoon garlic powder
1 tablespoon light miso paste slurry (or 1/2 teaspoon salt + 1 teaspoon soy beans or soy powder), to
    taste/health
1/8 teaspoon kala namak (egg flavor)

PREPARATION

* Add cashews (and cauliflower, if using) to a saucepan with 1/2 cup water, cover and bring to a simmer.
  Remove from heat, do not drain, let set 30 minutes to soak, then transfer to a blender and blend to a
  creamy consistency.
* Add remaining ingredients and blend all until creamy and smooth, adding a little water if needed.

Sour Cream

This makes about a cup and lasts for about a week in the refrigerator.

INGREDIENTS

1/2 block or 7-ounces unfrozen firm pressed tofu
2 tablespoons fresh blended lemon juice
2 tablespoons vinegar (rice vinegar or white balsamic work well)
1-2 teaspoons light miso paste, optional
1 teaspoon honey

PREPARATION

* Combine all ingredients in a blender and blend until creamy and smooth. Add a little water if needed.

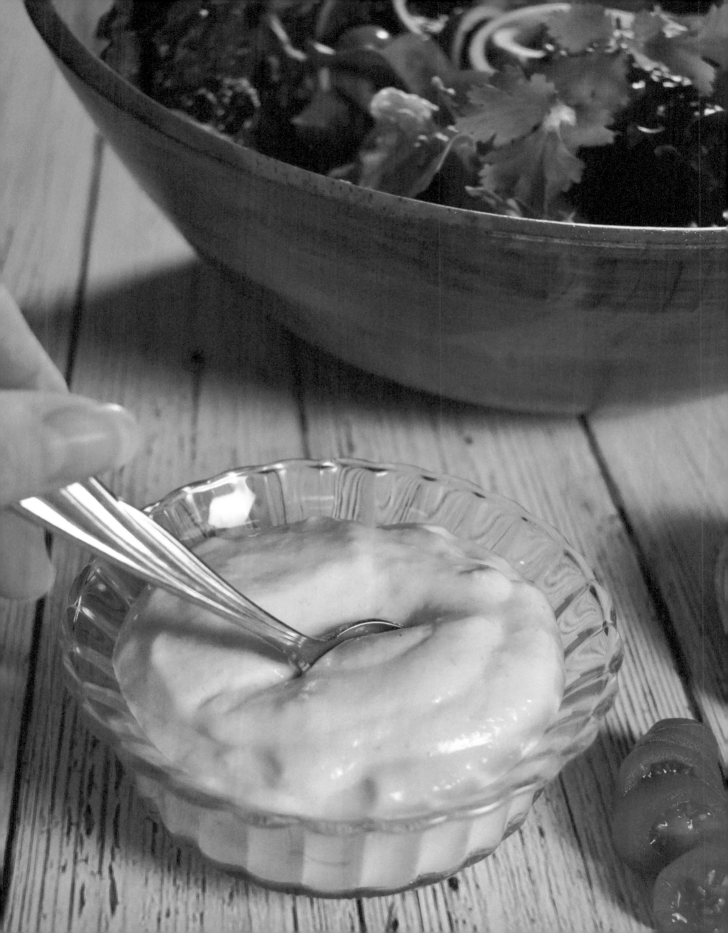

Red Curry Paste

Thai Red Curry is one of our favorite dishes that we discovered during our travels to Phuket, Thailand. This replacement curry does not have fish or fish oil in it as others often do. It is quite easy to add the healthy nutrients that seaweed has to offer with the same delicious flavor.

INGREDIENTS

4-8 red chili peppers or 1/2 cup (soak in water 10 minutes if dried)
1 tablespoon miso paste or 1/4 teaspoon salt, to taste/health
2-3 garlic cloves
2 tablespoons shallot or other mild onion
1 tablespoon lemongrass core, thinly sliced against the grain
1-2 tablespoons cilantro (stems and leaves)
1 tablespoon ginger root or galangal, minced
1/2 kaffir lime skin/peel, or 1 teaspoon regular lime zest/peel
2 teaspoons white pepper
1/2 teaspoon cumin powder
1/2 teaspoon coriander seed or powder

PREPARATION

* Place all ingredients except for white pepper, cumin, and coriander powder in mixer or blender and blend to thin paste, then transfer to a small bowl.

* Add remaining dry ingredients. and mix to a thick paste.

Milk, Cream, Cheese, Baked Goods

Oat Milk

Oat Milk Creamer

Soy Milk

Almond Milk

Parmesan Cheese

Ricotta Cheese

Cheddary Cheese Sauce

Cream Cheese

Bread Loaf

Pizza Crust

Flatbread

Oat Milk and Creamer

Many kinds of store-bought milk are fortified with calcium and other vitamins to help ensure that even those with poor diets get the minimum required nutrients, but it is best to get your calcium from your greens and other plants. Be sure you are eating a proper whole food plant-based diet or supplementing as needed. This milk is mildly sweet, creamy and delicious in coffee, tea, on cereal, in your oatmeal, and as a cold, creamy glass of milk anytime.

INGREDIENTS

5 cups water, divided (use much less water for creamer, adjust to taste)
1 cup of rolled oats
1 teaspoon of vanilla, optional
2 tablespoons date paste/syrup, pure honey, or maple syrup, optional

PREPARATION

* Place 2-3 cups of water and oats in a blender, and blend on high for 1-2 minutes.

* Taste and add more water to desired taste/consistency

* Drink as is or strain through a loose cheesecloth and transfer to a pitcher or container.

* Add vanilla and sweetener, to taste/health

Oat Creamer Powder for On the Go

Oat milk creamer found at some favorite coffee shops can be steamed up beautifully for a delicious, creamy, healthy dairy alternative. You can make your own oat milk creamer at home by finely blending oats into a powder with a coffee bean grinder or a blender and adding water. Unfiltered oat powder may leave a sediment in the bottom of your cup that can be enjoyed as a healthy treat. Place some powdered oats in a baggie to take with you anywhere to stir into to your coffee or tea—a great way to add creaminess and the fantastic healthy benefits of oats.

Soy Milk

INGREDIENTS AND SUPPLIES

1 cup dried soybeans (must be soaked overnight and boiled), can order organic soybeans online
1-2 tablespoons pure maple syrup or honey, optional to taste/health
Cheesecloth

PREPARATION

* Rinse soybeans well, drain, and add to a bowl with enough water to cover them by about an inch. Soak the beans for at least 10 hours, changing water every few hours, if possible.
* After soaking, change water and boil gently for about 30 minutes, drain, pour beans into a blender, add 4 cups of water, and blend until smooth.
* Pour soybean mixture through a cheesecloth or dishtowel over a pot to strain the milk. Repeat if desired with 2 more cups of water.
* In a pot on medium-high heat, bring soy milk to a boil for about 3 minutes, stirring and scraping sides and scooping to remove foam.
* Add 1-2 tablespoons sweetener and whatever flavor(s) you wish, such as vanilla, cocoa, banana, etc. Enjoy your homemade almond milk hot or cold.

Almond Milk or Creamer

INGREDIENTS

1 cup raw almonds, simmered and soaked
4-6 cups water (much less water for creamer)
1-2 teaspoons of vanilla, optional
1-2 tablespoons pure honey, date syrup, or maple syrup, optional to taste/health

PREPARATION

* Simmer and soak almonds for 30 minutes, drain water, add to a blender with another cup of water, and blend to a creamy butter.
* Add 3 more cups of water, and blend for a few more minutes. Add more water for desired consistency.
* If your blender works well, you can drink the almond milk "whole" or strain through a cheesecloth.
* Add honey, date syrup, or maple syrup, and blend until smooth.

Cheese Replacements

Commercial nondairy cheese products like shredded cheddar, mozzarella, and feta are available in many grocery stores. There is a wide array of ingredients in store bought products. They can be made from cultured nuts, seeds, and soy and may also contain refined oils and other unnatural ingredients. Compare labels to determine which ones contain the most whole plant-based ingredients. Here are some of the healthiest homemade sources to get you started.

Parmesan Cheese

This takes all of a minute or two to make. Consider adding it to an empty commercial parmesan cheese container. If you use nuts and there is a risk to someone you know with a nut allergy, be sure to add a label. For our family, this was one of the first cheese replacements we tried and enjoyed. We use it on pizza, pasta, and popcorn. You can use any combination of nuts or seeds in this and enjoy a wide array of nutrients.

INGREDIENTS

2 cups any combination of raw cashews, raw hemp seeds, raw shelled sesame seeds, pumpkin seeds, or
    sunflower seeds (my favorite is a combination of cashews and hemp seeds)
1/2 cup nutritional yeast
1/2 - 3/4 teaspoon salt, to taste/health
1 teaspoon soy powder to help buffer salt (See recipe)
1 teaspoon garlic powder
1/2 teaspoon onion powder

PREPARATION

To blend, add to a food processor, and pulse to a coarse powder, then stop. Overblending causes clumping and creaming. Raw hemp seeds may not need to be blended.

Ricotta Cheese

This recipe makes about 2 3/4 cups of ricotta that can be used as thin layers in lasagna.

1 ½ cups cashews, simmered, soaked, and drained or 1 ½ cups firm tofu, or cooked potatoes
1 cup cauliflower (chopped and steamed) or 1 cup white beans
1/4 teaspoon oregano, dried or 2 tablespoons fresh parsley, finely chopped
1 tablespoon lemon juice
2-3 tablespoons nutritional yeast
2 tablespoon honey or maple syrup (less with sweet cashews)
2 cloves garlic, minced or 1/4 teaspoon garlic powder
1 tablespoon light miso paste or 1/4 teaspoon salt + 1/2 teaspoon soy powder or soybeans/tempeh
1/4 tsp xanthan powder, optional for thickening
1 tablespoon parsley, finely chopped or 1/2 teaspoon dried

PREPARATION

Prepare and add ingredients to a food processor, and blend until creamy.

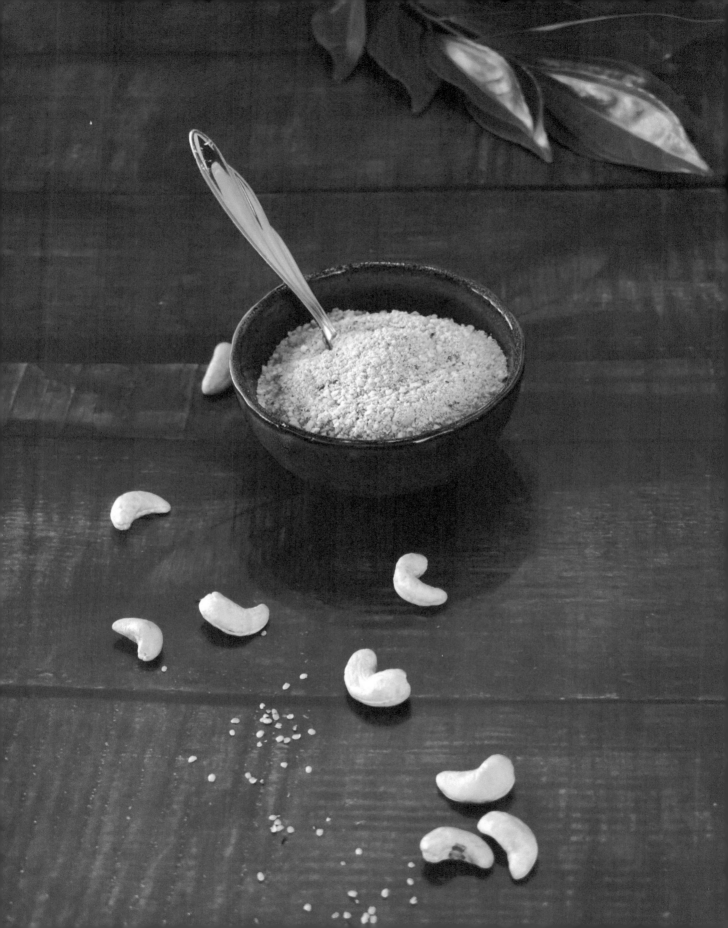

Cheddary Cheese Sauce

INGREDIENTS
1/2 cup cashews, 1/2 cup potatoes, or 1/2 cup white beans
1/2 cup cauliflower, chopped
1/3 cup carrot, 1/4-inch slices
1/4 cup onion, sliced
1 cup low sodium vegetable stock, broth, or water

OTHER INGREDIENTS
1 tablespoon lemon juice
1/2 teaspoon Dijon mustard
2 tablespoons light miso paste
1/2 teaspoon salt, to taste/health
1 teaspoon soy powder, tempeh, or soybeans to help buffer salt (See recipe)
1 pinch teaspoon celery seed
1/3 cup nutritional yeast
1/2 teaspoon garlic powder
1/8 teaspoon turmeric or paprika
1 dash cayenne pepper

PREPARATION
* Place INGREDIENTS in a saucepan over medium heat, cover, bring to a simmer for 5-7 minutes, cover with a lid, remove from heat, and allow to steam for 20 minutes. Do not drain.
* Transfer simmered/steamed ingredients to a blender, add OTHER INGREDIENTS, and blend until creamy. Adjust thickness with low sodium vegetable broth or water.

Cream Cheese

INGREDIENTS
1/2 cup raw soaked cashews, 1/2 cup potatoes, or 1/2 cup white beans
1 cup cauliflower, chopped and steamed
1/2 cup water

OTHER INGREDIENTS

2 tablespoons apple cider vinegar
2 tablespoons lemon juice
2 teaspoons honey
3 garlic cloves, minced, or 1/2 teaspoon garlic powder
1/2 teaspoon salt + 1 teaspoon soy powder, soybeans, or tempeh, to help buffer salt

PREPARATION
* Place INGREDIENTS in a saucepan over medium heat, cover, bring to a simmer for 5-7 minutes, cover with a lid, remove from heat, and allow to steam for 20 minutes. Do not drain.
* Transfer simmered/steamed ingredients to a blender, add OTHER INGREDIENTS, and blend until creamy. Adjust thickness with nondairy milk, low sodium vegetable broth, or water

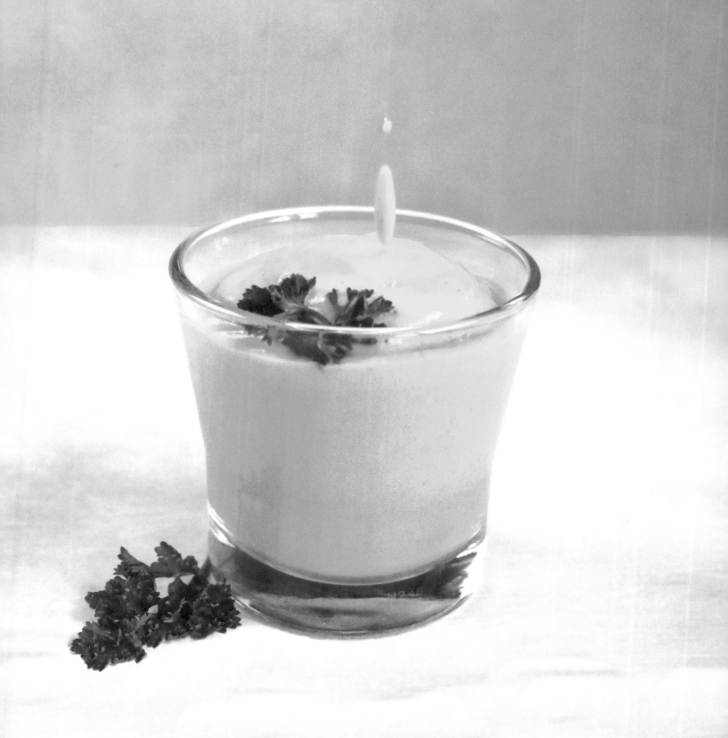

Baked Goods

Whole Grain Bread Loaf, Pizza Crust, and Flatbread

This amazing and very easy recipe is adapted from Rip Esselstyn' wife, Jill Esselstyn and is found in his cookbook, *Plant-Strong* which is a fantastic collection of hearty plant-based recipes. His interest in cooking healthy plant-based food developed through the work of his father, Dr. Caldwell Esselstyn, Jr. whose amazing research in reversing heart disease has saved thousands of lives. Rip noticed that a large number of his fellow firefighters shared variety of health problems, including heart disease and diabetes. He challenged them to try plant-based food and reversed their disease. His news spread throughout the country and he now has his own line of healthy food called Engine2 found at Whole Foods and many other stores. This dough can be made and kept in the refrigerator for about 10 days. Grab a piece to bake whenever you are ready for the great smell and taste of nutritious homemade bread.

INGREDIENTS

1 1/2 cups lukewarm water
1 1/2 cups unsweetened almond, rice, or soymilk, lukewarm
4 1/2 teaspoons or 2 packets of fresh granulated yeast
2-3 teaspoons natural salt, to taste/health,
5-6 tablespoons date sugar or pure cane sugar, to taste/health (for pizza crust consider using less)
1 tablespoon soy powder (or blended tempeh or soybeans) to help buffer salt
6 1/2 cups whole grain flour (whole grain pastry flour, optional)

PREPARATION

* Preheat oven to 350°F. Baking temperatures vary. See below

* In a large bowl, combine lukewarm water, lukewarm milk, yeast, salt, and sugar.

* Combine flour and soy powder and add to other ingredients in large bowl and combine using hands

* Coat with a little more flour to reduce stickiness, if needed.

* Allow the dough to set at room temperature for 2 to 3 hours to rise, then break off desired amount, form into the shape desired, allow dough to rise 30 minutes more, then bake (when using refrigerated bread, form into desired shape and allow 1 1/2 hours more rising time.)

* Bake time is anywhere from 8-10 minutes for muffin size on up to 60 minutes for cantaloupe-sized dough portions for loaves. Watch closely for light browning.

Sandwich Bread Loaf or Garlic Bread—Preheat oven to 350°F. Lightly coat desired amount of dough with flour and place it on a nonstick baking mat, in a nonstick loaf pan/mold or lightly sprayed loaf pan, or on parchment paper. For refrigerated dough, allow for 1 ½-hours re-rise time. Less rise time for warmer dough.

Cinnamon Raisin Bread—Same directions as above except flatten ball of dough to 1/2 inch, and layer it with 1/3 cup or more raisins and a good amount of cinnamon and nuts, as desired. Gently press raisins and nuts into dough and roll up into a loaf. Allow dough to rise another 45 minutes and if dough is cold, allow it to rise 1 ½ hours. Bake at 350°F for 50-60 minutes.

Pizza Crust—Preheat oven to 425°F. Sprinkle cornmeal on a pizza stone or on a pizza pan. Same directions as above except use grapefruit sized ball of dough. No need to allow re-rise. Flatten dough out 1/4-inch thickness. Bake 5-10 minutes to lightly brown. Top with pizza sauce, pesto, or white cream sauce, desired vegetables, and add a light layer of nondairy mozzarella and parmesan cheese (See recipe). Bake for about 20 minutes. Consider olives, onions, bell peppers, pickled peppers, spinach, and mushrooms.

Flatbread—Preheat oven to 300°F. Sprinkle nondairy parmesan or cornmeal on a preheated iron skillet or pizza stone. Add an orange- or grapefruit-sized piece of dough and flatten it out to about 1/4-inch thickness and transfer the pan to the oven for 10 minutes. This is delicious basted with a thin coating of nondairy butter and nondairy parmesan cheese, and garlic, dipped in balsamic vinegar, or used as an addition to a meal with pasta.

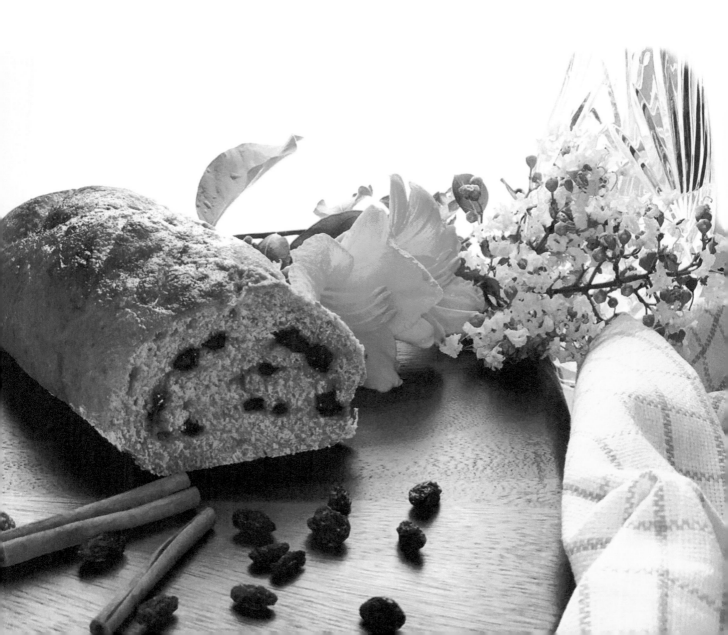

Cornbread or Corn Muffins

INGREDIENTS
1 1/2 cups cornmeal
1/2 cup whole grain flour
1 teaspoon baking powder
1/2 teaspoon baking soda
1/2 teaspoon natural salt + 1 teaspoon soy powder (or blended soybeans or tempeh)
1/2 teaspoon dried cardamom
1/2 teaspoon tarragon
3/4 cup fresh corn, roughly chopped or whole kernel
1/2 cup unsweetened applesauce or pumpkin purée
1/3 cup date sugar and pure cane sugar mix
1 3/4 cups unsweetened nondairy milk

PREPARATION
* Preheat oven to 350°F.
* Combine all ingredients.

Baking options and baking times:

* Line a nonstick baking dish, 9 x 9 inch with parchment paper on the bottom and bake for 20-25 minutes or until toothpick comes out clean in center.

or

* Pour into nonstick mini muffin cups and bake for 8-10 minutes or until edges are lightly browned.

Appetizers and Snacks

Health Boosted Guacamole

Favorite Salsa or Pico

Deviled Potatoes

Pineapple Salsa

Ceviche

Seven Layer Dip

Homemade Popcorn

Health Boosted Guacamole

I've used this recipe for decades. Over that time, I've learned to add beans, chickpeas, edamame, or green peas to reduce the fat and increase the nutritional value.

INGREDIENTS

3 avocados, chopped

3/4 cup edamame, peas, spinach, or beans, precooked or steamed and cooled

1 tablespoon lime juice

1/4 cup red onion or 1/2 cup sweet onion, chopped

3 cloves garlic, minced, pressed, or sliced

1/2 teaspoon ground pepper

10 sprigs cilantro, chopped, stems included

1 tablespoon pickled jalapeño juice

10 pickled jalapeño slices, chopped

1 small tomato, chopped, or 1/4 cup salsa

1-2 fresh serrano or jalapeño peppers, adjust to heat/spice preference

PREPARATION

* Add all ingredients to food processor and pulse-chop for chunky dip, stopping to stir under large chunks. Avoid turning to a purée, unless you prefer that consistency.

* Seal guacamole without air pockets to preserve color longer.

* Serve with low or unsalted whole grain chips, celery sticks, carrot sticks, raw bell pepper strips, air fried French fries, as a taco garnish/topping, or as a sandwich spread.

Favorite Salsa or Pico

MAIN INGREDIENTS

4-5 cups tomatoes, roughly chopped into a strainer to remove extra juice (use vine ripe when possible)

1/3 cup onion, sweet and/or purple, roughly chopped

2-3 tablespoons pickled jalapeño peppers, roughly chopped (our secret ingredient)

2 cloves garlic, minced

1/2-1 cucumber, chopped into small cubes, optional

DRESSING

2 tablespoons pickled jalapeño juice

1 tablespoon lemon juice

1 tablespoon light miso paste

1/4 teaspoon fresh ground pepper

PREPARATION

* Add all Main Ingredients to a food processor and pulse-chop to a chunky consistency, then transfer to a colander/strainer to drain excess water, allowing it to drain for at least 5 minutes.

* Transfer Main Ingredients to a mixing bowl and add Dressing.

* Toss to combine and serve with organic whole grain or organic corn chips.

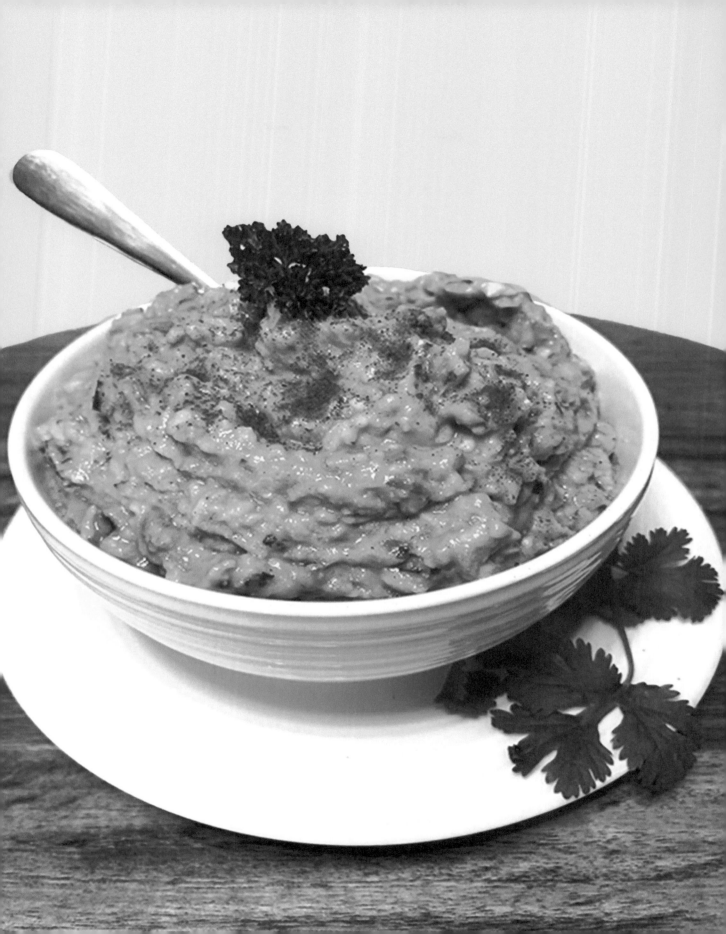

Deviled Potatoes

This lovely recipe idea was inspired by Ann and Jane Esselstyn, the wife and daughter of Dr. Caldwell Esselstyn, Jr. Many of my patients and relatives from western Pennsylvania farm country love cookouts and are deviled-egg lovers. Kala namak has an amazing egglike flavor.

POTATO "EGG WHITES" INGREDIENTS
10 small oval potatoes for "egg white shells," Makes 20 "deviled eggs" halves (see *PREPARATION* below)

PREPARATION FOR POTATO "EGG WHITES"
* Wash whole potatoes and place in microwaveable dish. Cover and microwave on high for 4 minutes.
* Remove potatoes from the microwave, allow them to cool to the touch, slice in half lengthwise, cut a flat sliver off the backside to help set potatoes level on a plate/platter, or place in egg tray or on serving dish.
* Heat large skillet or pot to medium-high with about 3/4 inch water. Place potatoes in it, cover, and cook for 8-10 minutes, until somewhat tender. Check with knife tip. Don't overcook. Rinse with cold water.
* Use a melon ball scoop or teaspoon to scoop out a large well from each potato half. Place scooped out potato in the food processor with other "egg yolk" ingredients.
* Place potato halves in the refrigerator to cool for 15 minutes.
* Use a spoon or a pastry bag to fill each potato half or "egg white" shell.

"EGG YOLK" INGREDIENTS
3 cups white beans or chickpeas
6 tablespoons plant-based mayonnaise (recipe available)
1 teaspoon Dijon or ground mustard
1/2 teaspoon lemon juice
3/4 teaspoon black salt/egg flavor/kala namak
1/2 teaspoon turmeric
1/4 teaspoon garlic powder
2 tablespoons sweet or dill pickle relish (add last)

PREPARATION FOR "EGG YOLKS"
* Combine *EGG YOLK INGREDIENTS*, except relish, in a food processor, and pulse to a creamy consistency.
* Add 2 tablespoons sweet pickle relish and pulse a couple times or hand stir to mix.
* Transfer yolks to a bowl or a pastry bag, and place in refrigerator for 15 minutes
* When shells are ready, use a spoon or a pastry bag to fill them.

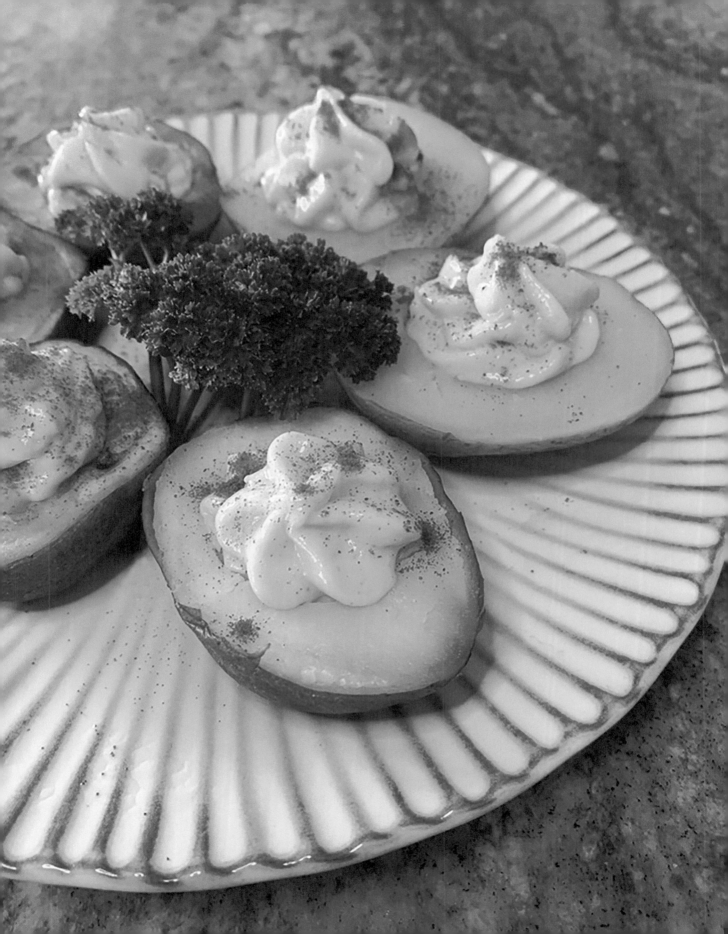

Pineapple Salsa

Using a whole pineapple, lay it on its side and slice the upper 1/3 away by first using knife to cut and oval shape, then use a large spoon to remove and hollow out, being careful not to puncture fleshy skin. Allow about a 1/2 inch of thickness to contain juices.

INGREDIENTS

1 cup diced pineapple
1 cup diced bell peppers, yellow, orange, or green
1 cup diced Roma, grape, or cherry tomatoes
1/3 cup chopped cilantro
1/4 cup red onion, chopped
2 limes juiced or 4 tablespoons lime juice
1/4 teaspoon black pepper or 1/16 tsp cayenne pepper, optional
1-2 jalapeño or serrano peppers
1/2 teaspoon cumin, optional

PREPARATION

In a large bowl, mix all ingredients, pour into pineapple, and serve with whole grain chips.

Ceviche

This is a popular and delicious appetizer in the Blue Zones of Costa Rica. Hearts of palm are a healthy dietary addition that can help reduce inflammation, lower blood sugar levels, improve digestive health and bone health, enhance weight loss, and improve immunity.

INGREDIENTS

1 jar hearts of palm, drained and chopped into pieces
1-2 tablespoons seaweed-nori, crushed or 1/8-1/4 teaspoon kelp powder
1/4 cup red onion, finely chopped
1 garlic clove, minced
1 cup bell pepper, orange, yellow, or green
1 cup cherry or grape tomatoes, diced
1 cucumber, diced
1/2 cup lime juice
2 teaspoons medium miso paste
1/4 cup cilantro, chopped
1/8-1/4 teaspoon ground black pepper
2 jalapeños, finely chopped, optional
2 avocados, cubed/chopped

PREPARATION

* In a medium bowl, combine all ingredients except for avocado.

* Toss to combine, then add the avocado by gently folding it into the other ingredients.

* Serve with whole grain tortilla chips or as a salad topping over greens.

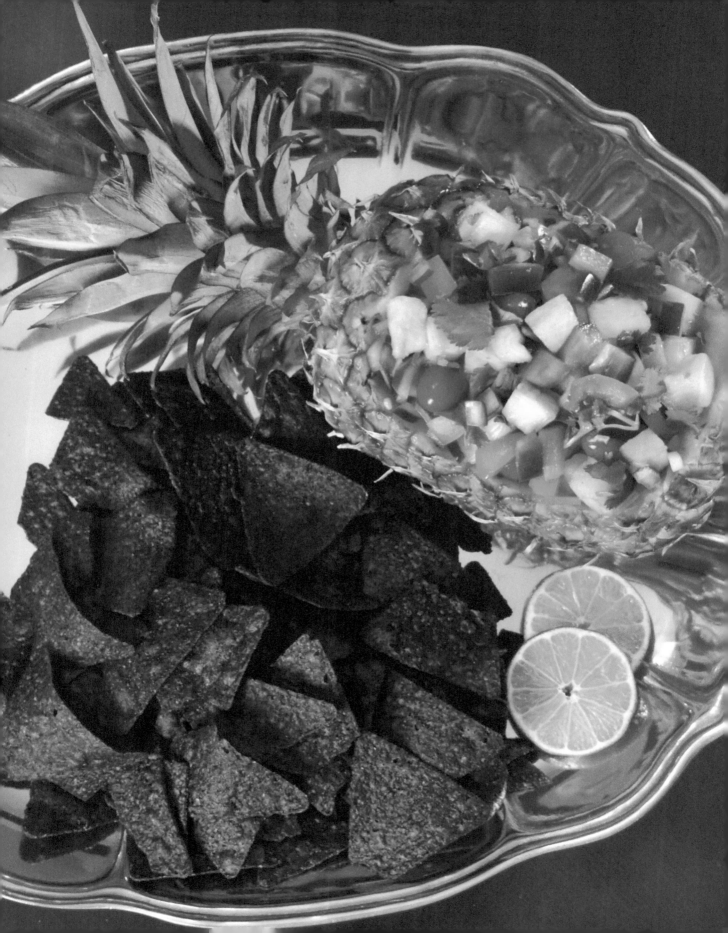

Seven Layer Dip

UNFRIED BEANS INGREDIENTS

2 cups pinto beans or a combination with other beans
1 tablespoon miso paste or low sodium soy sauce
1/4 teaspoon pepper
3 medium ripe avocados, mashed
1 tablespoon lime juice
1/2 teaspoon garlic powder
1 teaspoon miso paste or 1/4-1/2 teaspoon salt, to taste/health
1/2 cup "sour cream"
2 teaspoons "taco seasoning"
3/4 cup shredded "cheddar cheese" or "cheese" sauce
1 cup black olives, sliced or chopped
2 medium tomatoes, finely chopped or salsa
1 bunch or 1/2 cup green onions, chopped
1/2 cup fresh cilantro

PREPARATION

* Spread each layer as listed below in a glass casserole dish about 9 x 13 inches.

* Top with fresh cilantro.

* Chill for at least an hour or overnight.

    First layer—on the bottom of the dish—in a food processor, blend beans, miso paste, and pepper to a lumpy paste, adjust with a little water
    Second layer—avocado, lime juice, garlic powder, and miso blended in a food processor or mashed to combine
    Third layer—sour cream and taco seasoning mixed together (See recipe)
    Fourth layer—"cheddar cheese" or "cheese" sauce (See recipe)
    Fifth layer—olives
    Sixth layer—tomatoes or salsa
    Seventh layer—green onions

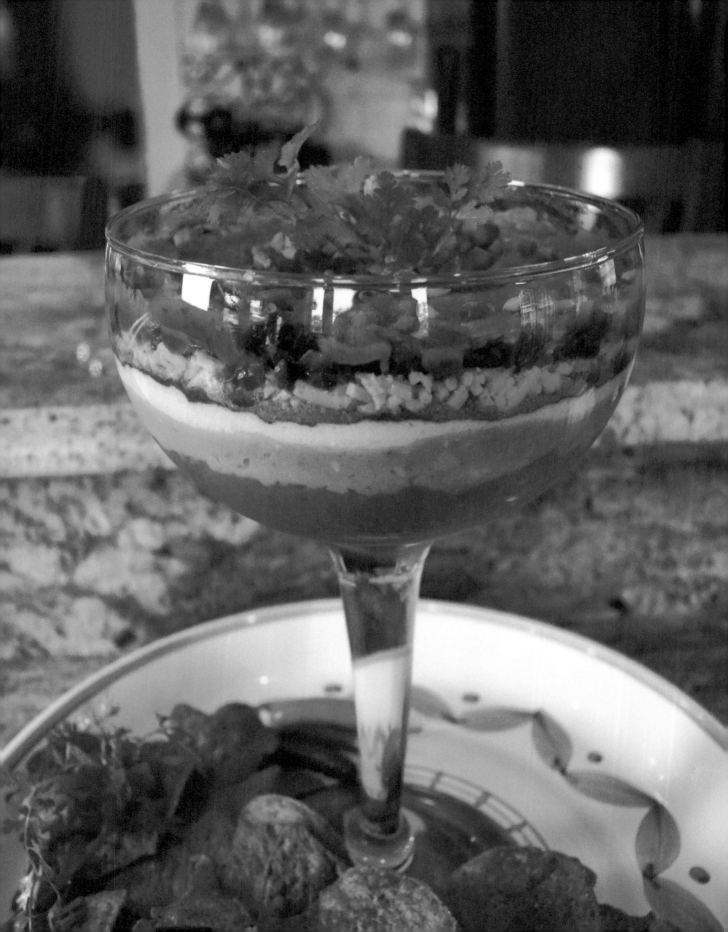

Homemade Popcorn

Many people enjoy popcorn, but most store brands are loaded with all kinds of unhealthy chemicals. You can easily make your own that can be a much healthier treat and much less expensive.

INGREDIENTS

1/2 cup organic popping corn
1 teaspoon nutritional yeast
2 teaspoons melted plant-based butter, optional
1/4 teaspoon salt + 1/2 teaspoon soy powder, optional

PREPARATION

* Add popcorn to a brown paper lunch bag, and fold over about ½ inch two times and press to flatten. Lay the bag with flap facing down in the microwave.

* Set microwave for 2 ½ minutes to cook and listen for early slowing of the popping sounds to stop.

* Transfer popped corn to a bowl, and place remaining unpopped corn back into the microwave for additional increments of time.

* Sprinkle or drizzle popcorn with desired topping.

Smoothies And Fruit Drinks

Vanilla Smoothie

Chocolate Smoothie

Cantaloupe/Pineapple Orange Slushy

Banana Berry Smoothie

Watermelon Slushy

Cucumber Pear Nojito

Hot Cocoa

Smoothies can be made with frozen, thawed, or fresh ingredients, but half-frozen and half-fresh works best. Be sure to keep a stock of peeled bananas in a baggie in the freezer to use as the base sweetener. Smoothies are a great way to start your day, and they make a wonderful anytime snack. To use frozen fruit and vegetables, lay them out for about 15 minutes before blending.

Vanilla Smoothie

Another delicious and healthy, go-to fix to have on hand.

ADD THE FOLLOWING TO A BLENDER:
1 banana, semifrozen
1 teaspoon vanilla paste, vanilla bean powder, or extract
1/2-3/4 cup plain, nondairy milk
2 teaspoons crushed flaxseeds
1 tablespoon vanilla soy/bean powder, optional

Chocolate Smoothie

Unbelievably yummy! This is a wonderful, healthy, go-to fix to have on hand to satisfy cravings.

ADD THE FOLLOWING TO A BLENDER:
1-2 rounded tablespoons 100% cocoa or cacao
1 banana, semifrozen
1/2 avocado optional for a creamier healthy addition
1/4 cup blueberries, optional for additional antioxidants
1/2-1 teaspoon vanilla bean powder, vanilla paste, or extract
3/4-1 cup nondairy milk
2-3 teaspoons crushed flaxseeds (or chia seeds)
1/2 cup kale or spinach
1 tablespoon vanilla soy/bean powder, optional
For a nutty twist, and more nutrients, add nuts or tahini

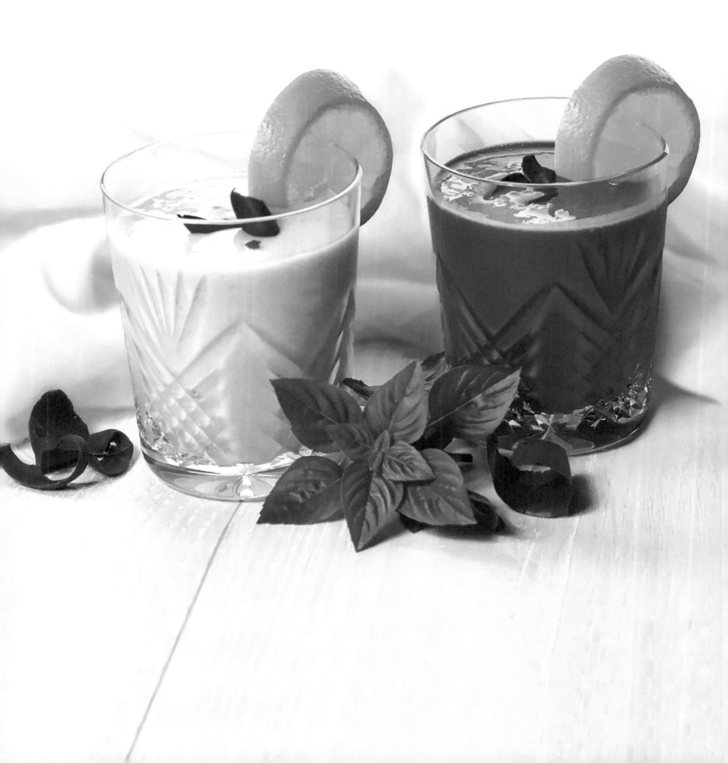

Cantaloupe or Pineapple Orange Slushy

A very impressive summertime or anytime treat. Cut cantaloupe or pineapple into pieces and freeze when perfectly juicy and ripe. This is a great way to prevent the waste of delicious healthy fruit.

INGREDIENTS
2 cups or 2 peeled fresh oranges with pith/fiber
1 ½ cups frozen cantaloupe pieces

PREPARATION
* Allow frozen cantaloupe to partially thaw for ten to fifteen minutes and add to a blender.
* Blend to a creamy-slushy consistency.
* Garnish with fresh basil, mint leaves, cantaloupe, or orange slice, optional.

Banana Berry Smoothie

This is a tasty treat that incorporates those important leafy greens and omega oils, not to mention mega antioxidants into your daily regimen decreasing dryness, enhancing that healthy glow, and improving your immune system.

ADD THE FOLLOWING TO A BLENDER:
1 banana, semifrozen
1 cup fresh or semifrozen blueberries and strawberries
1/2-3/4 cup leafy greens
1/2 peeled orange or 1 cup pineapple pieces, optional
1 tablespoon flaxseed or chia seed
1 cup nondairy milk or water

PREPARATION
Blend to desired consistency

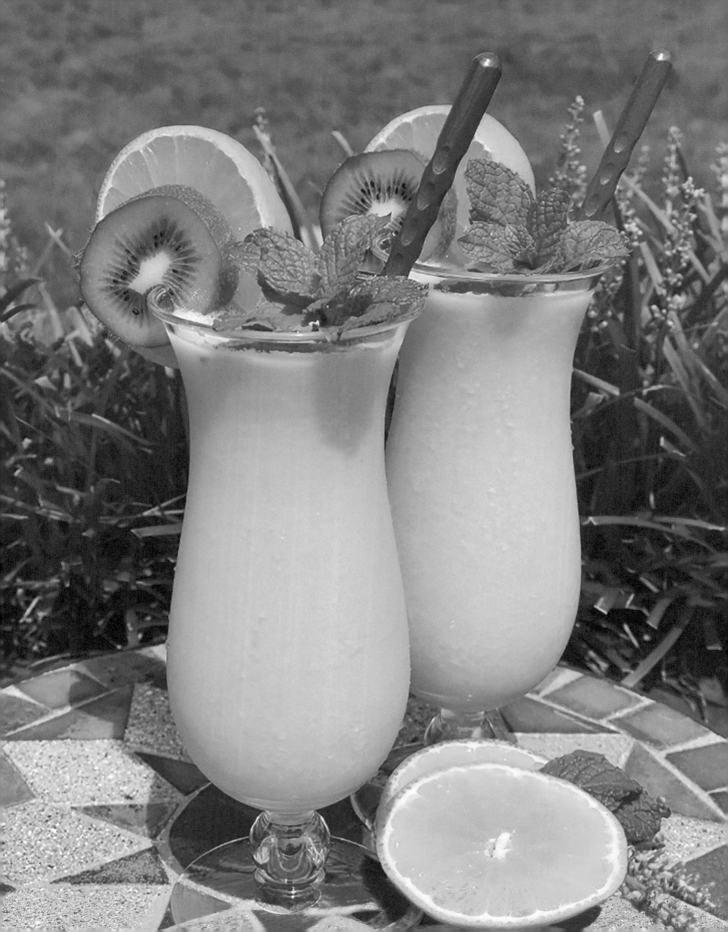

Watermelon Slushy

This is an ultimate summer or anytime treat. Cut watermelon into pieces to freeze and enjoy year round.

INGREDIENTS
Prefrozen watermelon cubes

PREPARATION
* Allow frozen watermelon to partially thaw for about ten minutes.
* Blend to a slushy consistency.
* Garnish with fresh basil, mint leaves, a slice of cucumber, or watermelon, optional.

Cucumber Pear Nojito

INGREDIENTS
1 cup prefrozen ripe pears (canned pears work also)
1 medium fresh or prefrozen cucumber
1 apple, peeled, unsweetened apple sauce (or soda water-add last, after blending)
4 mint or stevia plant leaves, add last after blending (roughly chopped)
1 tablespoon lime juice
1 cup water

PREPARATION
* Add ingredients to a blender (except soda and mint leaves) and blend to a slushy consistency.
* Garnish with fresh mint leaves, lime wedge, or cucumber sliced round.

Hot Cocoa

INGREDIENTS
1 rounded tablespoons cocoa
1-2 tablespoons maple syrup, honey, or date syrup
1 cup nondairy milk
1/4 teaspoon vanilla, optional

PREPARATION
* Add cocoa and syrup to a cup, stir with a spoon until creamy, then add milk and vanilla and stir.
* Microwave for a minute or two.

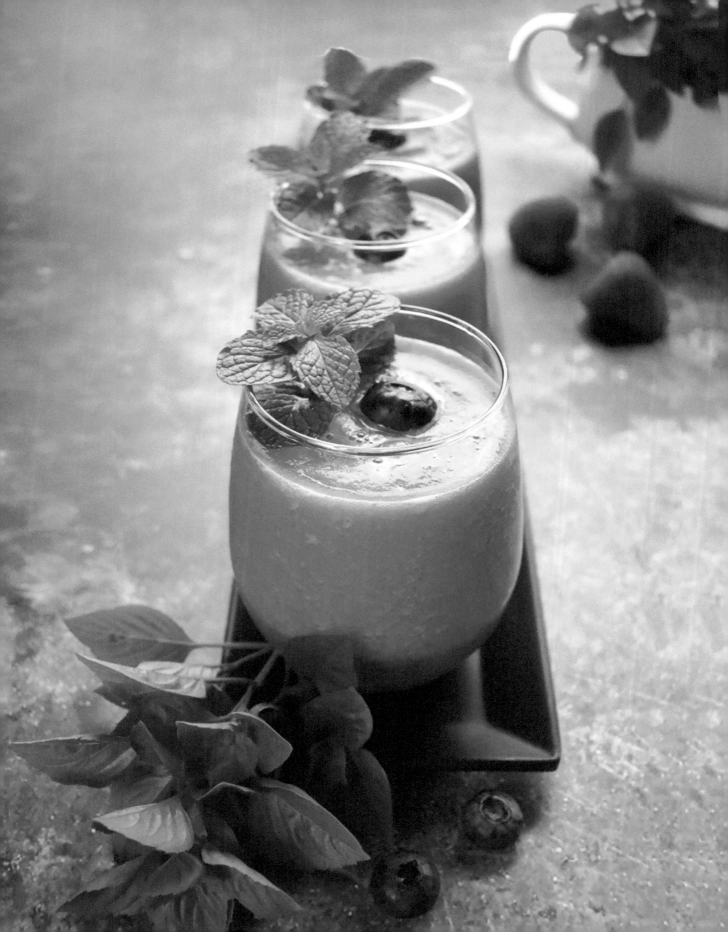

Desserts

Fruit Compote

Cocoa Bites

Brownies

Chia Pudding

Chocolate Chip Cookies

Banana Ice Cream

Vanilla Ice Cream

Chocolate Mousse

An important thing to remember about natural sweeteners: Your body uses only so much of them, then converts and stores the extra as fat in places you don't want it. This does not mean you can't have any, you just have to limit the amount you eat or work off the extra with exercise.

Fruit Compote

Fruit compote is another very healthy and delicious way to enjoy your fruit. It is basically a fruit jam or preserve, but with a much lower glycemic index (lower sugar) and no high fructose corn syrup. You can double this and make it to last a week or so, then use it anytime, cold or warmed, on or in anything such as oatmeal, pancakes, toast, chia pudding, or any other dessert. Frozen berries are picked when they are perfectly ripe and nutrient rich. Strawberries, peaches, blueberries, raspberries, kiwi, blackberries, cherries, and pears are all great options. For garnish, use berries, kiwi, raisins, mint, coconut flakes, lemon, orange, or lime zest.

INGREDIENTS

2 ½ cups fresh or frozen fruit (thawed)
1/4 cup of water
1-3 tablespoons date sugar, maple syrup, or honey, optional, depending on sweetness of fruit
2-3 teaspoons crushed chia seeds or flaxseed, thickener (can also consider ½ - 1 teaspoon xanthan gum)

PREPARATION

* Add ingredients to a blender and adjust to desired taste.

* Transfer to a saucepan over medium heat and bring to a simmer for a minute or two, stirring constantly.

* Remove from heat and allow to cool for 15 minutes, transfer to jars with lids or pour over dessert or other food and enjoy.

Cocoa Bites

These are so easy to make and a very impressive treat for sharing. No baking required.

COCOA BALL INGREDIENTS

14-16 dates, seeded
2 teaspoons flaxseed, crushed
1/3 cup chickpeas, finely chopped walnuts, or ¼ cup tahini
3-4 tablespoons pure cocoa powder
1/2-1 teaspoon vanilla powder, paste, or extract
1/2 teaspoon lemon juice
1/4 teaspoon cinnamon

COCOA BALL COATING OPTIONS

Cinnamon mixed with some date sugar or cane sugar. Cocoa powder, coconut flakes, chia seeds, or hempseeds spread out on plates.

PREPARATION

* Slice dates around their midsection, flip open and pluck out the seeds.
* Rinse dates, add to a food processor along with the remaining COCOA BALL INGREDIENTS, and blend well to a crumbly paste.
* Using your hands, roll mix into balls, then roll them in your choice of coating.

Brownies

Inspired by Dr. Greger from his book *How Not to Die*. Allergy friendly with seed replacment options. Another easy treat with no baking required.

INGREDIENTS

1 cup walnuts or hemp seeds
1 1/2 cup pitted dates
1/2 cup tahini or almond butter
1/2 cup cocoa powder
1/2 cup crushed pecans or pumpkin seeds

PREPARATION

* Add walnuts or hemp seeds and dates to a food processor and chop until finely ground.
* Add tahini or almond butter and cocoa and pulse to combine.
* Transfer mix to an 8" nonstick baking dish or baking mold, bottom lined with parchment paper.
* Using parchment paper on the top to prevent sticking, press mixture evenly into the pan.
* Peel away parchment paper, add crushed pecans or pumpkin seeds, lay paper over again and press into brownies, cover and refrigerate for an hour before cutting.

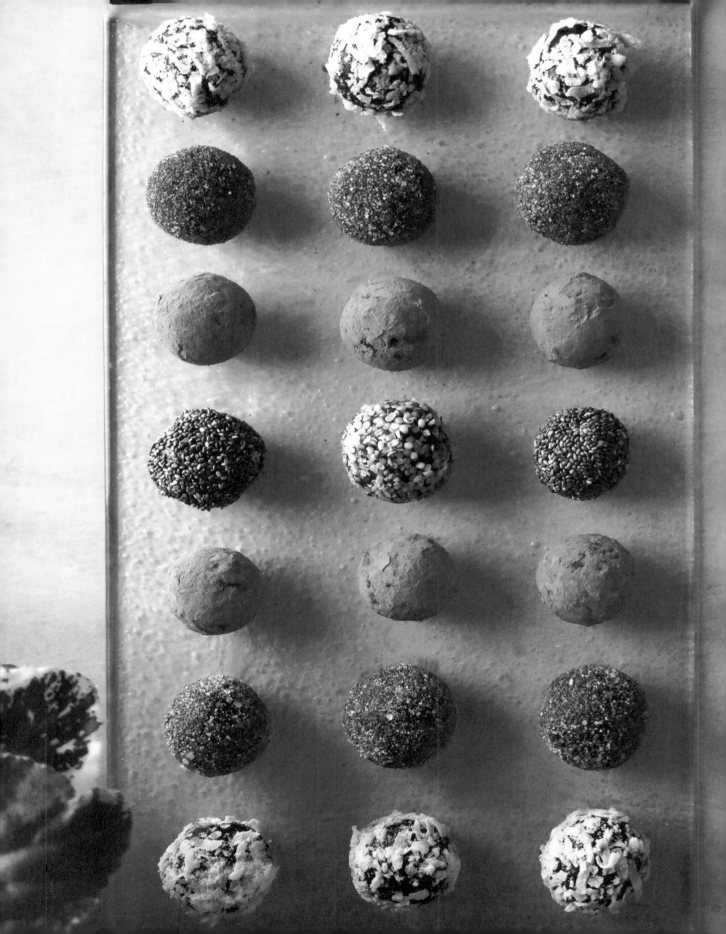

Chia Pudding

Chia seeds are packed with fiber, omegas, antioxidants, and protein. Chia seed pudding is probably the easiest, healthiest, and most common plant-based dessert you can make. Chia pudding is commonly served with fruit for breakfast as well. It is quite impressive to serve to guests with the colorful blended fruit and layers, garnished with berries, orange, lime or kiwi wedges and mint, seeds, nuts, cinnamon, coconut flakes, chocolate chips, or granola (maple pecan shown).

Many people love the texture of plump whole chia seeds, but chia seeds don't release much of their nutrients in that form. A combination of blended and unblended chia seeds can provide nutrients and fiber and add the texture many people love. A little date syrup, date paste, honey, or maple syrup make this a really tasty treat, especially for enticing children. For richer, creamier pudding and/or natural sweetness, add banana, silken tofu, avocado, nut butter, seed butter, or even lowfat coconut milk and xanthan powder for lighter color and thicker consistency.

INGREDIENTS

1 cup nondairy milk (for lighter color pudding, add additional milk and 3/4 - 1 teaspoon xanthan powder for each cup)

1/4 cup chia seeds, a mix of blended and unblended

1-2 tablespoons pure date syrup, honey, maple syrup, or blended fruit (banana, pineapple, or apple), adjust to taste/health

1 teaspoon vanilla extract

Fruit Compote for layering or as a topping, if desired (See recipe)

PREPARATION

* It takes less time for blended chia seeds to fully swell and thicken as a pudding. Heated chia seeds will plump up in about 15 minutes. Unheated chia seeds take at least 2 hours or overnight to fully plump.

* For compote layers, refrigerate between layering.

* To color chia pudding milk base, blend milk with some fruit like strawberries or blueberries and chia seeds.

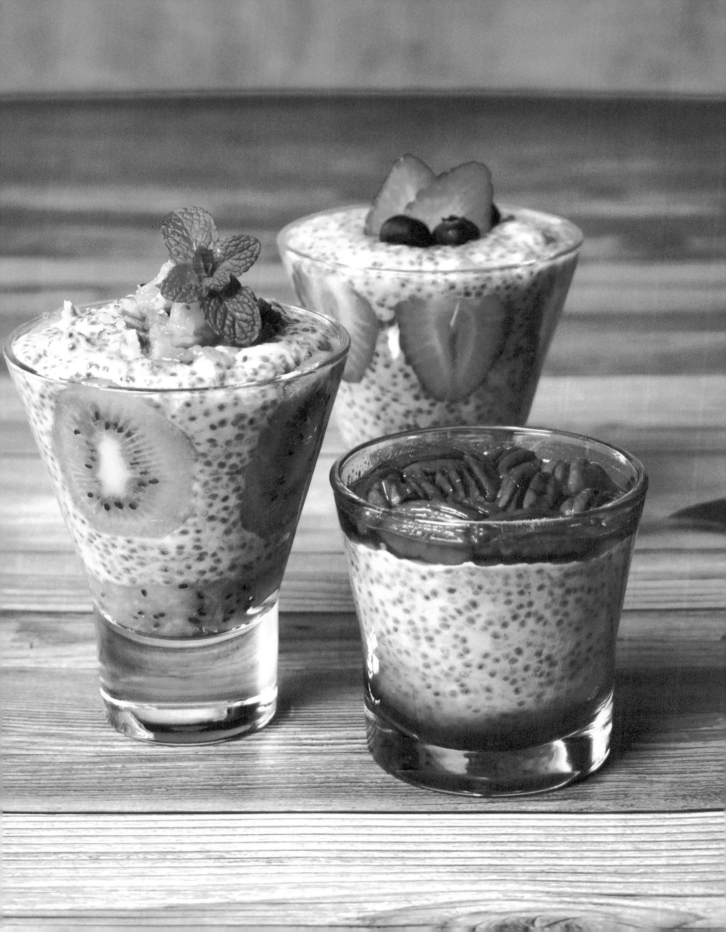

Chocolate Chip Cookies

These cookies are made by modifying "America's favorite cookie recipe," but the ingredients are switched out with healthier, whole plant-based ingredients. Tahini (sesame seed butter) and apple sauce take the place of 1 cup of butter. These sources contain fiber, so the amount of flour in the recipe is reduced to compensate for dryness of the dough. The sugar is replaced with mostly date sugar, but for those who enjoy a little bit of crispness around the edges of their cookies, the dough can be lightly coated with some pure sugar cane (limit this source of sweetener as it is not a whole food and is of insignificant nutritional value).

For you cookie dough lovers: though very rare, there are concerns of flour contamination. To eliminate that concern, flour can be spread out on a baking mat and heated at 400 degrees for 3-5 minutes or placed in microwave for about a minute, or almond flour can be used instead. There is no raw egg to worry about, either. Dough is less sticky after refrigeration.

DRY INGREDIENTS

1 ¾ cups whole grain flour or a combination of flour and oats (reduced from 2 ¼ cups)
1 teaspoon baking soda
1 teaspoon salt + 1 teaspoon soy powder (or blended soybeans or tempeh) to help buffer salt

OTHER INGREDIENTS

1/2 cup seed butter (tahini), nut butter, ripe avocado, or banana (if banana flavor is acceptable)
1/2 cup apple sauce
2 flax eggs (2 tablespoon crushed flaxseed + 6 tablespoons water. Allow to set for 10 minutes to gel)
1 ½ cups date sugar and some pure cane sugar combined until palate adjusts to more date sugar. Date sugar is a whole food healthy sweetener whereas *pure* sugar cane contains very little remaining nutrients after molasses extraction and processing.
1 teaspoon vanilla
1 - 1 ½ cups plant-based semisweet chocolate chips (2 cups is excessive-isolated/imbalanced omega oil)
1 cup chopped walnuts or pecans, optional

PREPARATION

* Combine flax and water and allow to set 10 minutes to gel.

* Combine DRY INGREDIENTS in one bowl and combine OTHER INGREDIENTS, except for chips, in another.

* Combine all ingredients and refrigerate dough for about an hour to make dough less sticky and rolling and shaping cookies easier.

* Preheat oven to 350°F.

* Use some flour on your hands to make dough less sticky and roll easier and consider a light coating of pure cane sugar to add some crispness. Place uncooked cookie balls on a baking sheet and press to flatten them into a cookie shape before baking (the extra fiber makes them hold their shape)

* Bake cookies for 7-10 minutes or until lightly browned (depends on size of cookies)

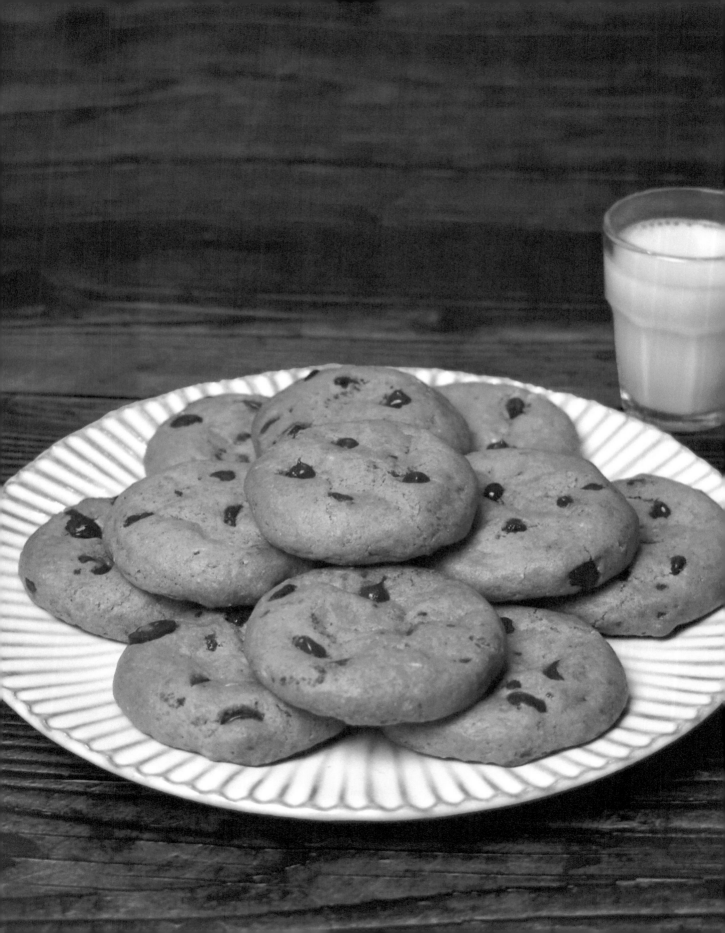

The creaminess of ice cream can be made from a blended, combination of frozen, semifrozen, and unfrozen whole plant ingredients such as bananas, nondairy milk, oat cream, lowfat coconut milk, cashew cream, or tahini. Sweeteners that have a low glycemic index and are high in fiber are dates, bananas, and berries. Other sweetening options include pure maple syrup, molasses, and natural honey. An ice cream maker or churn can make ice cream making fun. Guar gum is added to help prevent crystallization and enhance creaminess.

Banana Ice Cream

For soft serve ice cream, blend semifrozen ingredients to a soft serve ice cream consistency.

To reduce banana flavor, consider adding 2 tablespoons dry powdered oats and 1/4 cup nondairy milk or 1/2 cup raw cashews soaked and blended to a cream.

For firm, scoopable ice cream place soft serve in the freezer for about 3 hours.

FLAVOR OPTIONS:

* **Strawberry:** Blend 2 semifrozen bananas, 1-2 cups semifrozen strawberries, and 1/4 teaspoon guar gum (optional). Freeze for at least 2-3 hours.
* **Chocolate:** Blend together 2 semifrozen bananas, 1/4 cup nondairy milk, 1-2 tablespoons cocoa powder, 1/4 teaspoon vanilla bean powder, paste, or extract, and 1/4 teaspoon guar gum (optional). Freeze for at least 2-3 hours.
* **Salted Caramel:** Blend together 2 semifrozen bananas and freeze for 2 1/2 hours (1/4 teaspoon guar gum optional). Meanwhile, Blend 7 pitted dates, 1/3 cup warm water, and 1 1/2 tablespoon cocoa powder to make a cocoa swirl. Add a small amount of natural salt to swirl when ready to add to semifrozen banana blend and then continue to freeze for 2-3 more hours.
* **Mint Chocolate Chip:** Blend together 2 semifrozen bananas, 1/4 cup nondairy milk, 2 tablespoons powdered oats, 6-8 mint leaves, and 1/4 teaspoon xanthan gum. Blend well, then stir in or blend chocolate chips or cocoa nibs. Freeze for at least 2-3 hours.
* **Peanut Butter:** Blend together 2 semifrozen bananas, 1/4 cup nondairy milk, 2 tablespoons powdered oats, 2-4 tablespoons peanut butter or tahini, and 1/4 teaspoon guar gum (optional). Freeze for 2-3 hours.
* **Cookies 'n Cream:** Blend together 2 frozen bananas, 2 tablespoons powdered oats, 1/4 cup nondairy milk, and 1/4 teaspoon guar gum. Add 3-4 Oreo cookies chopped into small pieces. Freeze for 2-3 hours.
* **Chocolate Avocado Cream:** Blend together 2 semifrozen bananas, 2 tablespoons powdered oats, 1/4 cup nondairy milk, 1/2 avocado, 2 tablespoons cocoa powder, vanilla bean powder, paste, or extract, and 1/4 teaspoon guar gum (optional). Freeze for 2-3 hours.

Banana replacement options: 1 cup soaked and creamed cashews + 1/4 cup powdered oats + 1/2 cup lowfat coconut milk or nondairy milk.

Vanilla Ice Cream

Though bananas and Medjool dates are perhaps the healthiest way to sweeten your ice cream, there are those who just want creamy, classic plain vanilla ice cream. This is as close as I could comfortably get healthwise and tastewise. See if you can make it even better.

INGREDIENTS

1 1/2 cups nondairy milk
1/2 cup powdered oats, blended dry to a powder
1/2 teaspoon guar gum powder (combine with oats)
1/4 cup creamed cashews, tahini, or hemp seeds, well-blended to a cream, optional
1/2 cup lowfat coconut milk, optional
1/2 cup date paste, maple syrup, honey, or pure cane sugar, to taste/health
1 1/2 teaspoons vanilla bean powder, vanilla paste, or extract

PREPARATION

* Blend oats to a powder in a coffee grinder or dry blender and combine with guar gum powder.

* Add nuts or seeds to a blender and blend until creamy (seeds can take up to 10 minutes to cream).

* For semifrozen milk, add all ingredients to the blender on high for 1-2 minutes until creamy and enjoy as soft serve ice cream.

* For unfrozen milk, transfer to an ice cream churning machine for 35-40 minutes. If not using ice cream machine, add 1/3 cup portions to containers to freeze for up to 3 hours and remove from the freezer about 15 minutes before serving to allow some thawing and blend again if necessary.

* Top with your choice of fruit, fruit compote, date caramel, date fudge sauce, fresh fruit, nuts, or seeds. One or two crushed oreo cookies are a definite favorite for many (not whole food, of course).

Chocolate Mousse

Truly one of our favorites. When I made this with dairy sources, I had very little self-control limiting to 1 or 2 of these. Now I don't worry and can eat to my heart's content - quite literally!

INGREDIENTS

1 banana (sweetest option), 1 1/2 cups raw cashews (simmered and soaked), 1 cup tahini, or 1 avocado

10-12 dates pitted, simmered and soaked (slice around mid-section, flip lid, and remove seed). Adjust amount of dates used if using bananas.

1 block or 14 ounces of tofu (silken or firm, not previously frozen)

1/2 cup lowfat coconut milk, optional (leftover coconut milk can be used in smoothies)

2/3 cup pure cocoa powder

2 teaspoons pure vanilla bean powder, paste, or extract

3/4 cup date syrup, date paste, or maple syrup (adjust sweetness)

LAYERING INGREDIENT

Raspberry or mixed berry *Fruit Compote* (See recipe), optional

20-30 Oreos, crushed or blended for a tasty layer treat (nice presentation and fun for kids), optional

PREPARATION

* If using cashews, simmer in ½ cup of water for 5 minutes, then add dates, cover with a lid, soak/steam for 20 minutes more, and drain excess water.

* Add cashews (or banana, tahini, or avocado), dates, and ½ of the tofu to the blender and blend until creamy, scraping sides with a rubber spatula.

* Add remaining INGREDIENTS and blend on high until creamy and smooth (may want to consider transferring to a food processor, depending on size of blender).

* Consider adding other flavors to mousse like fresh mint or peanut butter, optional.

* Spoon into dessert or parfait glasses in layers and refrigerate for a couple hours or overnight.

* Garnish with raspberries, blueberries, orange slices, mint leaves, or shaved chocolate.

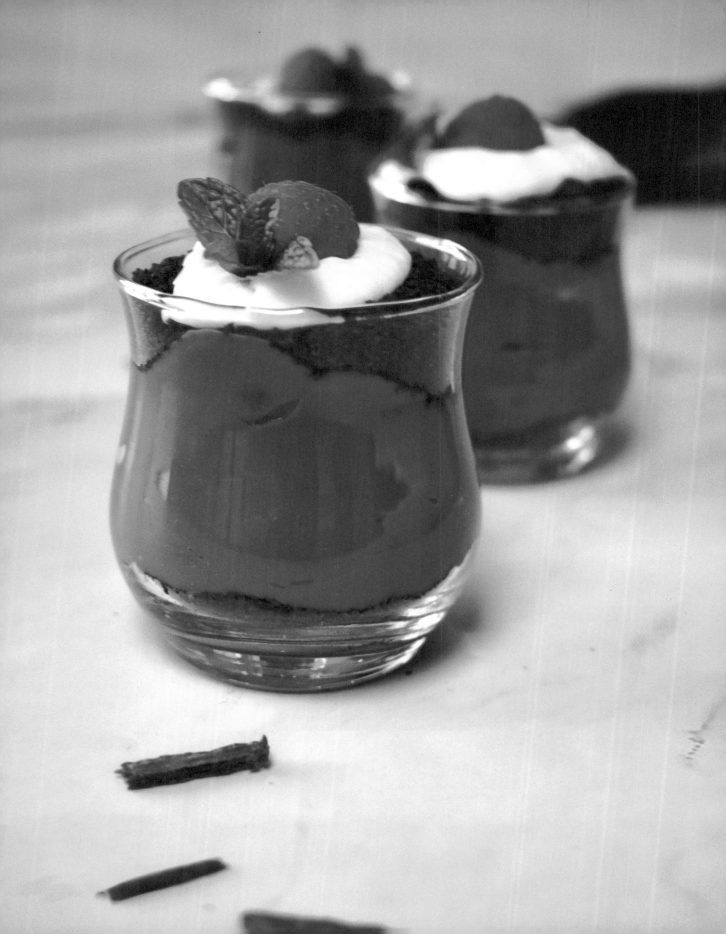

About the Author

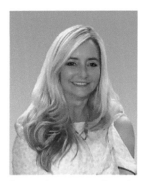

Pamela spent her growing years helping her family tend their gardens that provided them with plenty of natural healthy food year-round. These years are where her love of healthy plant food began. Having been raised near Annapolis, Maryland, Pamela met and married her military spouse in 1988 and spent nearly 30 years traveling and moving every couple years or so. Those years extended her experiences in unimaginable ways. While managing a nursing career, she had landed senior spouse roles with deploying combat squadrons and ships with families numbering from 200 to 5000. She shared responsibilities which included providing assistance, counseling, crisis management, morale boosting, catering, entertaining, and so much more for members from all over the world while all were separated from their core families.

Her journey included over twenty years practicing as a nurse caring for people in various settings and at all levels from intensive care in open-heart surgery, cancer, and neurology to management of patients in home care and hospice. She has worked in communities and hospitals all over the country. Pamela has seen firsthand how people in certain cultures beat the American longevity and health odds. While working as a nurse in various parts of California, she witnessed how differently many patients handled recovering from surgery. She noted that her hospice patients in Blue Zones were generally older, more alert, and had more functionality at end of life compared to other hospice patients she encountered in other parts of the country. It became apparent to her that their diet played a key role in their success. Through rigorous nursing assessments, observations, and discussions with patients and medical professionals, Pamela conducted personal research on the effect of food on her patients' health. In so doing, she has seen the damage food can cause inside and outside of the human body. She developed a strong belief that "food is thy medicine," and as a result, a strong passion for helping people establish healthy eating habits in order to extend and improve their lives. Her interest in this lifestyle led her to the discovery of the scientists who have spent more than 60 years fully immersed this amazing science and she continues to provide nursing care in her community with her firm belief that a Whole Food Plant-Based Lifestyle does in fact improve people's lives.

References

[1] N. I. o. Health, "Dietary Reference Intakes (DRIs): Recommended Dietary Allowances and Adequate Intakes, Vitamins and Elements," *National Academy of Pediatrics,* 2011 2011.

[2] M. Heron, "Deaths: Leading Causes for 2017," Online, National Vital Satistics Reports vol. 68, US Department of health and human services, CDC, p. 1, June 24, 2019.

[3] S. Ramkumar, A. Raghunath, and S. Raghunath, "Statin therapy: review of safety and potential side effects," *Acta Cardiologica Sinica,* vol. 32, no. 6, p. 631, 2016.

[4] E. L. Richman, S. A. Kenfield, M. J. Stampfer, E. L. Giovannucci, and J. M. Chan, "Egg, red meat, and poultry intake and risk of lethal prostate cancer in the prostate-specific antigen-era: incidence and survival," *Cancer prevention research,* vol. 4, no. 12, pp. 2110-2121, 2011.

[5] W. W. Tang *et al.*, "Intestinal microbial metabolism of phosphatidylcholine and cardiovascular risk," *New England Journal of Medicine,* vol. 368, no. 17, pp. 1575-1584, 2013.

[6] R. A. Koeth *et al.*, "Intestinal microbiota metabolism of L-carnitine, a nutrient in red meat, promotes atherosclerosis," *Nature medicine,* vol. 19, no. 5, pp. 576-585, 2013.

[7] G. E. Dunaif and T. C. Campbell, "Relative contribution of dietary protein level and aflatoxin B1 dose in generation of presumptive preneoplastic foci in rat liver," *Journal of the National Cancer Institute,* vol. 78, no. 2, pp. 365-369, 1987.

[8] T. C. Campbell, "Dietary protein, growth factors, and cancer," *The American journal of clinical nutrition,* vol. 85, no. 6, pp. 1667-1667, 2007.

[9] C. B. Esselstyn Jr, S. G. Ellis, S. V. Medendorp, and T. D. Crowe, "A strategy to arrest and reverse coronary artery disease: a 5-year longitudinal study of a single physician's practice," *Journal of Family Practice,* vol. 41, no. 6, pp. 560-568, 1995.

[10] T. C. Campbell, B. Parpia, and J. Chen, "Diet, lifestyle, and the etiology of coronary artery disease: the Cornell China study," *The American journal of cardiology,* vol. 82, no. 10, pp. 18-21, 1998.

[11] J. Wick, "Diverticular disease: eat your fiber!," *The Consultant Pharmacist®,* vol. 27, no. 9, pp. 613-618, 2012.

[12] M. J. Orlich *et al.*, "Vegetarian dietary patterns and mortality in Adventist Health Study 2," *JAMA internal medicine,* vol. 173, no. 13, pp. 1230-1238, 2013.

[13] B. F. O. K. Wendel. "Plant-based diet vs. Vegan diet: What's the difference:." https://www.forksoverknives.com/wellness/plant-based-diet-vs-vegan-diet-whats-the-difference/ (accessed June 13, 2020).

[14] P. J. Tuso, M. H. Ismail, B. P. Ha, and C. Bartolotto, "Nutritional update for physicians: plant-based diets," *The Permanente Journal,* vol. 17, no. 2, p. 61, 2013.

[15] J. Ruzzin and D. R. Jacobs, "The secret story of fish: decreasing nutritional value due to pollution?," *British Journal of Nutrition,* vol. 108, no. 3, pp. 397-399, 2012.

[16] E. P. o. C. i. t. F. Chain *et al.*, "Risk for animal and human health related to the presence of dioxins and dioxin-like PCBs in feed and food," *EFSA Journal,* vol. 16, no. 11, p. e05333, 2018.

[17]   C. Bergkvist *et al.*, "Dietary exposure to polychlorinated biphenyls is associated with increased risk of stroke in women," *Journal of internal medicine,* vol. 276, no. 3, pp. 248-259, 2014.

[18]   M. Greger. "The Risks of Fish Oil Supplements." https://nutritionfacts.org/2018/02/20/the-risks-of-fish-oil-supplements/ (accessed).

[19]   D. Rodriguez-Leyva *et al.*, "Potent antihypertensive action of dietary flaxseed in hypertensive patients," *Hypertension,* vol. 62, no. 6, pp. 1081-1089, 2013.

[20]   M. Greger. "This Week's Power Food: Flax Seeds." https://nutritionfacts.org/audio/this-weeks-power-food-flax-seeds/ (accessed January 10, 2020).

[21]   M. Greger. "Why is Milk Consumption Associated with More Bone Fractures?" https://nutritionfacts.org/2017/01/31/why-is-milk-consumption-associated-with-more-bone-fractures/ (accessed January 20, 2020).

[22]   M. Greger. "Iodine Supplements Before, During and After Pregnancy." https://nutritionfacts.org/video/iodine-supplements-before-during-and-after-pregnancy/ (accessed).

[23]   R. Russell *et al.*, "Dietary reference intakes for vitamin A, vitamin K, arsenic, boron, chromium, copper, iodine, iron, manganese, molybdenum, nickel, silicon, vanadium, and zinc," *A Report of the Panel on Micronutrients, Subcommittees on Upper Reference Levels of Nutrients and of Interpretation and Uses of Dietary Reference Intakes, and the Standing Committee on the Scientific Evaluation of Dietary Reference Intakes Food and Nutrition Board Institute of Medicine,* 2001.

[24]   J. Hever, "Plant-based diets: A physician's guide," *The Permanente Journal,* vol. 20, no. 3, 2016.

[25]   S. Ziaei and R. Halaby, "Dietary isoflavones and breast cancer risk," *Medicines,* vol. 4, no. 2, p. 18, 2017.

[26]   X. O. Shu *et al.*, "Soy food intake and breast cancer survival," *Jama,* vol. 302, no. 22, pp. 2437-2443, 2009.

[27]   M. Greger. "The Difference Between Alpha and Beta Receptors Explain Soy's Benefits." https://nutritionfacts.org/2020/03/24/the-difference-between-alpha-and-beta-receptors-explain-soys-benefits/ (accessed January 2020).

[28]   M. Greger. "Is Miso Healthy?" https://nutritionfacts.org/video/is-miso-healthy/ (accessed 2019)).

[29]   K. Ito, K. Miyata, M. Mohri, H. Origuchi, and H. Yamamoto, "The effects of the habitual consumption of miso soup on the blood pressure and heart rate of Japanese adults: a cross-sectional study of a health examination," *Internal Medicine,* vol. 56, no. 1, pp. 23-29, 2017.

[30]   C. Nagata, N. Takatsuka, N. Kawakami, and H. Shimizu, "Soy product intake and hot flashes in Japanese women: results from a community-based prospective study," *American Journal of Epidemiology,* vol. 153, no. 8, pp. 790-793, 2001.

[31]   M. Greger, "Beer Phytoestrogens," 2019. [Online]. Available: https://nutritionfacts.org/2019/06/04/beer-phytoestrogens/.

[32]   M. Greger. "Cut the Calorie Rich and Processed Foods." https://nutritionfacts.org/video/cut-the-calorie-rich-and-processed-foods/ (accessed 2020)).

[33] M. Greger. "Food as Medicine: Preventing and treating the most common diseases with diet." https://www.youtube.com/watch?v=d0IhZ-R1O8g&t=1429s (accessed).

[34] W. J. Craig and A. R. Mangels, "Position of the American Dietetic Association: vegetarian diets," *Journal of the American Dietetic Association,* vol. 109, no. 7, pp. 1266-1282, 2009.

[35] K. A. Mulder, D. J. King, and S. M. Innis, "Omega-3 fatty acid deficiency in infants before birth identified using a randomized trial of maternal DHA supplementation in pregnancy," *PLoS One,* vol. 9, no. 1, p. e83764, 2014.

[36] M. R. Flock, W. S. Harris, and P. M. Kris-Etherton, "Long-chain omega-3 fatty acids: time to establish a dietary reference intake," *Nutrition reviews,* vol. 71, no. 10, pp. 692-707, 2013.

[37] J. A. Greenberg, S. J. Bell, and W. Van Ausdal, "Omega-3 fatty acid supplementation during pregnancy," *Reviews in obstetrics and Gynecology,* vol. 1, no. 4, p. 162, 2008.

[38] D. R. Jacobs Jr, J. Ruzzin, and D. H. Lee, "Environmental pollutants: downgrading the fish food stock affects chronic disease risk," *Journal of internal medicine,* vol. 276, no. 3, pp. 240-242, 2014.

[39] A. C. o. Obstetricians, Gynecologists, and C. o. H. C. f. U. Women, "Committee Opinion No. 496: at-risk drinking and alcohol dependence: obstetric and gynecologic implications," *Obstetrics and gynecology,* vol. 118, no. 2 Pt 1, p. 383, 2011.

[40] G. Carson *et al.*, "Alcohol use and pregnancy consensus clinical guidelines," *Journal of obstetrics and gynaecology Canada,* vol. 32, no. 8, pp. S1-S2, 2010.

[41] D. Pascali-Bonaro, "Childbirth education and doula care during times of stress, trauma, and grieving," *The Journal of Perinatal Education,* vol. 12, no. 4, pp. 1-7, 2003.

[42] M. Greger. "Is Type 1 Diabetes Triggered by the Bovine Insulin in Milk?" https://nutritionfacts.org/2019/11/28/is-type-1-diabetes-triggered-by-the-bovine-insulin-in-milk/ (accessed).

[43] J. Strong and H. McGill Jr, "The pediatric aspects of atherosclerosis," *Journal of atherosclerosis research,* vol. 9, no. 3, pp. 251-265, 1969.

[44] Y. M. Hong, "Atherosclerotic cardiovascular disease beginning in childhood," *Korean circulation journal,* vol. 40, no. 1, pp. 1-9, 2010.

[45] C. B. Khambatta, R,. "The Incredible Benefits of a Plant-Based Diet for People with Type 1 Diabetes." https://www.forksoverknives.com/wellness/plant-based-diet-benefits-for-type-1-diabetes/ (accessed 2019)).

[46] N. D. Barnard, A. R. Scialli, G. Turner-McGrievy, A. J. Lanou, and J. Glass, "The effects of a low-fat, plant-based dietary intervention on body weight, metabolism, and insulin sensitivity," *The American journal of medicine,* vol. 118, no. 9, pp. 991-997, 2005.

[47] N. D. Barnard *et al.*, "A low-fat vegan diet and a conventional diabetes diet in the treatment of type 2 diabetes: a randomized, controlled, 74-wk clinical trial," *The American journal of clinical nutrition,* vol. 89, no. 5, pp. 1588S-1596S, 2009.

[48] R. J. Barnard, T. Jung, and S. B. Inkeles, "Diet and exercise in the treatment of NIDDM: the need for early emphasis," *Diabetes care,* vol. 17, no. 12, pp. 1469-1472, 1994.

[49] N. D. Barnard. "How to reverse diabetes in 3 steps." https://www.youtube.com/watch?v=SuwR46p7wrA&t=107s (accessed).

[50] M. Greger. "Is Gluten Sensitivity Real?" https://nutritionfacts.org/video/flashback-friday-is-gluten-sensitivity-real-separating-the-wheat-from-the-chat/ (accessed 2019).

[51] Physicians Committee for Responsible Medicine. "Everything You Need to Know About Gluten." https://www.youtube.com/watch?v=L2tLW2fiSqI (accessed).

[52] B. Dieter and R. Time, "The Gluten Manifesto: Everything You Need to Know About Gluten."

[53] J. Zheng, Y. Zhou, Y. Li, D.-P. Xu, S. Li, and H.-B. Li, "Spices for prevention and treatment of cancers," *Nutrients,* vol. 8, no. 8, p. 495, 2016.

[54] V. Bagnardi, M. Blangiardo, C. La Vecchia, and G. Corrao, "Alcohol consumption and the risk of cancer: a meta-analysis," *Alcohol Research & Health,* vol. 25, no. 4, p. 263, 2001.

[55] A. Britton, M. Marmot, and M. Shipley, "Who benefits most from the cardioprotective properties of alcohol consumption—health freaks or couch potatoes?," *Journal of Epidemiology & Community Health,* vol. 62, no. 10, pp. 905-908, 2008.

[56] R. J. Johnson, B. Rodriguez-Iturbe, T. Nakagawa, D.-H. Kang, D. I. Feig, and J. Herrera-Acosta, "Subtle renal injury is likely a common mechanism for salt-sensitive essential hypertension," *Hypertension,* vol. 45, no. 3, pp. 326-330, 2005.

[57] S. Yusuf, S. Reddy, S. Ôunpuu, and S. Anand, "Global burden of cardiovascular diseases: part I: general considerations, the epidemiologic transition, risk factors, and impact of urbanization," *Circulation,* vol. 104, no. 22, pp. 2746-2753, 2001.

[58] E. D. Freis, "The role of salt in hypertension," *Blood pressure,* vol. 1, no. 4, pp. 196-200, 1992.

[59] M. Guasch-Ferré *et al.*, "Nut consumption and risk of cardiovascular disease," *Journal of the American College of Cardiology,* vol. 70, no. 20, pp. 2519-2532, 2017.

[60] B. K. McFarlin, K. C. Carpenter, T. Davidson, and M. A. McFarlin, "Baker's yeast beta glucan supplementation increases salivary IgA and decreases cold/flu symptomatic days after intense exercise," *Journal of dietary supplements,* vol. 10, no. 3, pp. 171-183, 2013.

[61] M. Greger. "Benefits of Nutritional Yeast for Cancer." https://nutritionfacts.org/video/benefits-of-nutritional-yeast-for-cancer/ (accessed 2019)).

[62] M. Greger. "What About Coconuts Coconut Milk, & Coconut Oil MCTs?" https://nutritionfacts.org/video/what-about-coconuts-coconut-milk-and-coconut-oil-mcts/ (accessed 2019)).

[63] N. Neelakantan, J. Y. H. Seah, and R. M. van Dam, "The Effect of Coconut Oil Consumption on Cardiovascular Risk Factors: A Systematic Review and Meta-Analysis of Clinical Trials," *Circulation,* vol. 141, no. 10, pp. 803-814, 2020.

[64] E. Yu, V. S. Malik, and F. B. Hu, "Cardiovascular disease prevention by diet modification: JACC health promotion series," *Journal of the American College of Cardiology,* vol. 72, no. 8, pp. 914-926, 2018.

[65] N. Okarter and R. H. Liu, "Health benefits of whole grain phytochemicals," *Critical reviews in food science and nutrition,* vol. 50, no. 3, pp. 193-208, 2010.

[66] C. J. Seal and I. A. Brownlee, "Whole-grain foods and chronic disease: evidence from epidemiological and intervention studies," *Proceedings of the Nutrition Society,* vol. 74, no. 3, pp. 313-319, 2015.

Index